"I had been trying to change my diet for many years without success—I was often tired, drank coffee daily, had severe PMS, and carried an extra 10-15 lbs. . . . With each cleansing procedure I go through at the Koyfman Center, I have more energy . . ."
—*L.C.*

"I was pretty mixed up in my food choices. . . . Dr Koyfman's reasoning has begun to make sense for me of the things I have felt and struggled with for a lifetime. . . ."
—*W.Z.*

"I was not doing very well with my diet and had a lack of energy. My gall bladder was giving me terrible problems. . . . I went through the colon, small intestine, liver, stomach, lymph, and cell cleanses, which included a seven-day fast. I have never felt better. . . ."
—*S.S.*

Find the completion of these testimonials in the chapter near the end of the book entitled, "Testimonials."

Healing through Cleansing Diet

Book 4: Control Your Weight and Your Health—Naturally

Eating Simply,

Healthy and

Delicious . . .

by Dr. Yakov Koyfman, N.D.

Practical Guide to a Healthy Lifestyle

Dedication

This little book is dedicated to the idea

That cleansing one's body of the toxins we take in
(from our food, water and air)
is an essential pathway to optimum health;

That natural techniques,
which are gentle and powerfully effective,
can and do remove the majority of these toxins;

and

That properly practicing
simple everyday cleansing procedures
is an important element
in one's overall detoxification program.

This book is one in a four-part series entitled:

Healing through Cleansing.

Book 1 is about the cleansing of the main excretory organs, the colon, kidneys, lungs and skin.

Book 2 tells how to cleanse the organs located in the head and neck region, the brain, thyroid gland, eyes, salivary glands, ears, nose and sinuses, throat, tongue, teeth and gums.

Book 3 deals with cleansing the abdominal organs, the stomach, small intestine, liver, blood vessels and blood, lymph, sexual organs, joints and spine.

Book 4 presents the main principles of a healthy diet with simple recipes for preparing living food dishes and safe cooking techniques which help to prepare freshly cooked foods without losing vital nutrients. Includes a weight loss program.

Each of these books contain testimonials both in the beginning and at the end of the book.

Preface

This book is published not as a substitute for, but rather as a supplement to, the care of your professional healthcare provider. More specifically, the procedures described in this book are designed to support the body's immune system through cleansing specific internal organs and systems down to the cellular level. In this way the body can be freed from the toxins it has picked up over the years, and its natural healing capacity strengthened. The information and techniques in this book are preventative in nature for the improvement of human health.

The information and the techniques described in this book are *not* designed to provide medical consultation or advice, diagnosis, prognosis, treatment procedures or prescription of remedies for any ailment or condition as those terms might be defined or construed by any federal, state or local law, rule, regulation or ordinance. Specifically, this book is not intended to engage in anything that legally would constitute the practice of medicine. The author of this book does not claim to treat any disease or provide any cure.

Instead, the information in this book is designed to create a better understanding of how the human body is capable of taking in and/or storing various chemicals, waste products and unwanted biologic organisms that are detrimental to human health. Further, this book is designed to discuss the impact these have on the human body, and how their partial or complete removal is beneficial to your health. Additionally, by increasing your awareness of these processes, this book hopes to create a greater self-awareness of personal health.

Because each person is unique, the author encourages each reader to pursue a daily self-care program tailored to his or her particular situation, based on that person's own best evaluation of the circumstances and in consultation with his or her professional healthcare provider.

Contents

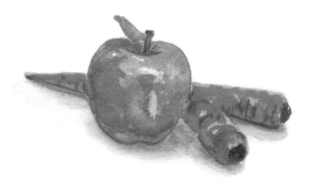

Introduction

Diet for Health

Young and healthy people don't always notice the relationship between diet and health. Youth carries with it a reserve of strength, but with age our reserves dwindle and those who are observant can notice that their well-being greatly depends on their diet.

On one hand, diet can supply the body with enzymes, vitamins, minerals, and proteins. On the other hand, it can poison the body.

One's diet can give energy or take it away. Diet can bring health or it can bring disease. So, what you eat is very important to your health. **If you master the art of proper eating, you will have the key to health in your hands.** In the world of nutrition there exist many different diets. Let me list just a few: macrobiotic, aurveda, Atkins, makers, vegetarian, vegan, raw food, living foods, blood type, and many more. Each of these diets insist on their own quality and downgrade the others. In some diets one product is considered healthy and nutritious, in others, the same product is a serious threat to your health. In most cases, authors who offer these diets begin in this approximate matter: "I was feeling so sick and began trying many different diets in order to improve my health. None of the diets helped me. Then I tried this diet and it worked like a charm. Now I am absolutely healthy and I recommend this diet to everyone."

Where Is the Author's Mistake?

One individual found a diet, which is perfect for him/herself. However, in other dieting systems, which did not work for that author, can be found many people for whom it worked amazingly. So each person has to find his or her own diet, which will work best for this person. To find the diet right for you, it is important to listen and understand the language of your body.

The first step to finding a contact with your own body is Cleansing of the Whole Body Organs and Systems from toxicity and parasites. Only then can your sensitivity increase to the point of feeling and understanding your body's language.

2

None of your organs or cells crave junk food. All they really want is nutrients. You may learn not only to understand which foods work best for you, but also to train your intuition to feel which nutritional product, depending on its particular nutrient mix, is needed in your system at the time.

Which Diet Should Be Considered Healthy?

A Real healthy diet is a diet that not only feeds the body, but also cleanses, heals, and strengthens it.

The dietary principles listed below are the chief guidelines for improving digestion and reinforcing your health. There are hundreds of various supplements for improving digestion, for cleansing the blood and all organs, for providing vitamins and minerals, for the immune system, and for other uses.

All of them can more or less make you healthier. However, that is ONLY if you follow all the fundamental dietary principles. If your diet is not correct, it does not matter what supplements you take. Instead of supplying your body with nutrients, you are poisoning yourself.

So, if you do not follow important principles of Healthy eating, described in my book "Healing Through Cleansing Diet," none of those systems will work effectively. By following the main principles of healthy eating, you develop a new dieting system—a "Cleansing Diet," which in itself combines all the best qualities of the systems listed above, and at the same time becomes **your Individual Diet.**

After you correctly pick out your individual diet and follow the main principles, which help the food to digest into nutrients, you have to make sure that those nutrients are able to be absorbed into your blood and delivered to the organs and cells. To make this process possible, it is necessary to cleanse and improve the function of your Small Intestine , where all the nutrient absorption takes place.

In the average person, small intestine's walls are covered with toxic mucus and toxic bile. Those layers stand in the way of nutrient absorption, depriving the body and weakening the immune system. In addition, 70-90% of all parasites, including unfriendly bacteria, yeast and other parasites, live and breed in the small intestine where they grab the nutrients first, even before the walls of your small intestine could absorb any nutrients into the blood.

You can completely cleanse your small intestine in our Center.

To learn more about unique cleansing procedures done in our center, please visit our website at
www.koyfmancenter.com

Principles of Healthy Eating

IMPORTANT NOTE:

If during your life time you allowed yourself to eat fast foods and sweets, drink coffee, eat late at night, and never followed any diet principles– it might be hard for you to change all of these harmful habits over night. However this should not disappoint or discourage you. Carefully learn the theory of principles provided in this book and start applying them slowly, step by step. This way you won't get overwhelmed and it won't seem impossible and difficult.

Start by changing one of your meals, for instance breakfast. Other two meals lunch and dinner may stay without changes. Changing only one meal of the day should not be of too much effort, especially if you carefully learn the principles of healthy eating and realize the importance of these changes. Without real knowledge and understanding, it would be much harder to do that.

When you get used to your new regiment, one to two weeks later you may change your lunch as well. Now you have two healthy meals a day and only one of what you are used to. In another couple of weeks, try to follow these principles all throughout one day staying away from all bad habits such as coffee, alcohol, fast food, snacks between meals, etc. The next day see how you feel.

Then try to have three "healthy" days in the row. If after that you have a strong urge to go back to your old eating habits–do so. Eat what you love and pay attention to how you feel after.

Gradually your bad cravings will start to diminish and your body will remember its nature and will ask for healthy foods more. However, if some days you feel that you want to eat something not very healthy, but psychologically pleasant and delicious for you–go ahead and do so. Very soon your body will start to understand what is good and what is bad for it. You will start noticing that your body is asking for healthy foods more frequently. Cleansing procedures described in my books "Healing Through Cleansing 1-3" and "Deep Internal Body Cleansing" would help the process and speed it up even more. Cleansing procedures will cleanse your digestive system from toxicity and parasites (which induce and provoke unhealthy cravings) and cleanse your digestive glands. When your digestive glands are cleansed, your taste preferences will go together with nature. You will begin to feel pleasure from eating healthy foods, eat less and feel better.

Those who are very ill, or who are ready to change, should make that change quicker or even immediately instead of gradually. When you are ready psychologically– challenge should not scare you off.

Principle 1. *Do Not Buy or Eat Industrially Processed Food*

You should buy natural, organic food, and prepare or cook it yourself. Industrially processed food loses part of the solar energy stored in it, along with a percentage of critical vitamins, minerals, and enzymes.

6

Principle 2. *Try to Buy Naturally Grown Food*

Organic or naturally grown food contains more nutrition and should not have any poisonous artificial chemicals. Some people say, "I'm eating a lot of fruit and vegetables and still don't feel good." They don't understand that if the fruit and vegetables are not organic, especially if used in large quantities, they can give a lot of toxins to the system and poison it.

Principle 3. *Try Not to Store or Preserve Food for Later Consumption Once It Is Prepared*

The chief principle here is to prepare or cook for one meal for immediate consumption. This principle allows you to receive the maximum amount of nutrients in their natural form. Food that spends 1-3 or more days in the refrigerator loses part of its nutrients and undergoes chemical changes for the worse.

Principle 4. *If You Have Good Digestion, Make Your Diet 75-100% Raw Food*

Vitamins, minerals, enzymes, etc., can be damaged or destroyed by cooking. Except for some foods such as meats which must be cooked, raw foods retain the maximum amount of the nutrition. When you must cook your food, do so in such a way that you would want to eat it. If you have poor digestion, you may prepare some of your food sparingly so that a minimum of the nutrients are damaged. You should consider eating foods raw if they do not form toxic gasses during digestion. This can include fresh vegetable juices and salads made of fresh cucumbers, tomatoes, carrots, etc.

Principle 5. *At Any Meal, Always Start Eating with Raw Salad or Raw Fresh Juices*

A dietician from Germany found that when cooked food touches the palate, the body treats it like a poison and sends a signal to the stomach to build up a defense. On the walls of the stomach white blood cells gather to suppress and neutralize the toxins of cooked food. This mobilization lasts for 1-1½ hours and then stops. If we eat cooked food 3-5 times a day, such mobilization of white blood cells keeps them from their most important work of defense thus weakening the body's immune system. This is one of the serious reasons why we get many diseases.

If we start eating any meal with fresh vegetables or fresh salad or fresh vegetable juice before eating something cooked, this situation will not happen. In this case, the immune system does not treat cooked food like a poison as it does when we start with it.

If you follow this rule, you may eat 10-40% cooked food (in the wintertime more than in the summer). This will do no damage to your system and allow you to keep some of your taste habits. You don't have to say good-bye to some of the cooked food that you love. Don't be a fanatic, refusing ever to eat anything cooked. We live in a real world and sometimes we need to eat cooked food when we socialize. Remember, eating cooked food will not damage your system if you practice moderation, begin with something raw, and do not overeat.

Principle 6. *Do Not Overeat*

This is one of the most important principles simply because if you choose to overeat even the best food it will bring more toxicity than nutrition. To understand how your stomach works when it is too full, you can do an experiment with a party balloon. Fill the balloon moderately with air and then let the air out. The balloon will easily return to its initial size. Now fill it as much as you can without popping it. You will notice that its walls have become thinner, and when you let the air out, it is no longer capable of returning to its normal state.

The walls of the stomach thin out during overeating, the stretched muscles weaken and can no longer churn the food as efficiently. An overfilled, stretched stomach presses against the liver, heart, lungs, and other organs. All these organs respond to the pressure by pressing back on the stomach. This resistance exhausts the organs. That is why after a large meal instead of the expected boost of energy we feel weak, tired, and sleepy.

Under the weight of too much food, the pyloric sphincter opens long before the food is properly digested. The undigested, unready food goes into the intestines, where instead of passing on nutrients through absorption, it begins the process of fermentation.

Why do we overeat? First, if we eat unsuitable, poor food that does not contain a good supply of nutrients, the blood never gives the signal of satiation, since such food does not contain what the cells need to live.

Second, if we eat good food, but swallow quickly without chewing, again the blood does not send the signal of satiation, or sends it only after a long time. Thus, eating too fast can also lead to overeating.

Third, many people eat under stress, losing all control over themselves. It is during stressful times that they eat sweets or other unsuitable food. This food is poorly digested and irritates the stomach walls. Next the person imagines that other food would calm this irritation. He or she eats other food, but calmness doesn't come, and he or she again opens the refrigerator in hope of finding something calming.

How can you prevent overeating? To do this, you should
- Supply the body with real nutrition, and
- Create the conditions for its quick absorption into the blood.

As you know, fluids are absorbed and get into the bloodstream faster than anything else. Liquids rich in nutrients include:
- Fresh juices of fruits and vegetables.
- Herbal tea.
- Vegetable decoctions.
- Ghee dissolved in tea.
- Extracts of greens and vegetables left overnight.
- Reconstitutions of dried fruits and vegetables.

If, 30-60 minutes before eating, you consume 1-2 glasses of such a drink, the nutrients will quickly enter the blood. By the time you start to eat solid food, the nutrients in the fluid will already have reached the bloodstream and cells. In this case, the satiation signal will come more quickly. This will go a long ways towards preventing you from overeating.

Most people have the habit of eating quickly. They swallow large, unchewed chunks and finish the entire meal in 5-10 minutes. This food, processed by neither the teeth nor the saliva, is difficult for the body to extract nutrients from, and the absorption of these chunks takes hours. Of course, the satiation signal does not come after 5-10 minutes, and the person, having filled the stomach, still feels hungry. Most people continue to eat, pushing the food into the overfilled stomach, stuffing it until other organs can no longer resist the pressure or until the food reaches the throat. Then they have to stop eating even though they may still not want to stop. If you chew each piece of food until the **solid food becomes liquid**, the food can then be more easily and more quickly digested. If you consume your normal meal slowly, over 30-40 minutes, the nutrients from the first portion of food consumed will get to the bloodstream, and the satiation signal will reach the brain before your stomach is overfilled.

Thus, to prevent overeating, you should drink a nutritious fluid 30-60 minutes before your meal and eat slowly, thoroughly chewing your food until it becomes liquid. Under these conditions, the satiation signal comes after only 30-40 minutes, and in a cleansed body faster still.

How much food can you eat in one meal without overeating? If you chew thoroughly, your body will give the satiation signal at the proper time on its own accord, and you do not need to weigh your food. Depending on your height and individual build the permissible amount of food to be consumed in one meal will vary.

Aurveda recommends that you eat as much as fits in both your hands held together.

How do you calculate your permissible amount of food per meal? Normally, the size of a person's internal organs depends on his or her height. Most likely, there is a dependence between the size of a person's organs and certain external features of that person, i.e., a person's heart is about the same size as his or her clutched fist.

The size of a person's normal, unstretched stomach is the same as the volume contained between his or her hands if held in the shape of a rectamgle.

A = B = Width of a hand.
C = Length of a hand.
V = AxBxC = Volume of the rectangle.

Example: If a person's hands are 7 cm. wide and 12 cm. long, then A = B = 7 cm., and C = 12 cm. To calculate the volume of the stomach, V = AxBxC = 7x7x12 = 588 cu. cm.

To convert measurements, 588 cu. cm. is about 600 gr. or 24 oz. Thus, 24 oz. or 3 glasses = the volume of this person's stomach.

This person should eat 2/3 of this volume per meal (16 oz. or 400 gr.) One third of the stomach must remain empty to accommodate the gases that form during digestion.

Principle 7. *Pay Attention to Food Combinations*

The major principles of proper food combination are:
• Do not mix fruits with anything else.
• Do not mix melons (including watermelons) with anything, including fruit.
• Do not mix protein and carbohydrates.

Poor combinations cause strong gas formation and waste a lot of energy for digestion. As a result, blood is poisoned with toxins and you feel weak and sleepy.

By following the principles of proper food combining you conserve food energy, prevent a variety of diseases and stabilize your weight.

Good combinations include:
• Starches and sprouts with vegetables.
• Protein and green leafy vegetables.

12

- Avocado and green leafy vegetables.
- Avocado and subacid fruit.
- **Poor combinations** include:
- Fruits and starches.
- Fruits and vegetables.
- Fruits and protein.
- Starches and protein.

The key to knowing the type of food lies in knowing its digestion time. Examples follow:

- **Proteins require 4 hours:** Nuts (almonds, pecans, walnuts), seeds (sunflower, sesame, pumpkin).
- **Starches require 3 hours:** Sprouted grains (wheat, rye, barley), sprouted legumes (chickpeas, lentils, peas), winter squashes, potato.
- **Vegetables require 2 ½ hours:** Sprouted greens (alfalfa, buckwheat, lentil, mung, sunflower), leafy greens (broccoli, cabbage, celery, kale, lettuce, spinach), fruit vegetables (cucumber, bell pepper, summer squash, zucchini).
- **Wheatgrass requires 15-30 minutes:** Use only on empty stomach or before meals. Extract juice by chewing or juicing. Use alone or with other vegetable juices.
- **Acid fruits requires 1–1½ hours:** Lemons, oranges, grapefruit, pineapple, strawberries, pomegranates.
- **Subacid fruits require 1½-2 hours:** Apples, pears, grapes, peaches, sweet cherries, apricots, kiwi, mango, most berries.
- **Sweet fruits require 4 hours:** Bananas, dried fruits (figs, dates, raisins), persimmons.
- **Melons require 15-30 minutes** and should always be eaten alone: Cantaloupe, crenshaw, honeydew, watermelon. When juicing, use the entire fruit, including rind.

(Source: Brian R. Clement, Theresa F. DiGeronimo, *Living Foods for Optimum Health.*)

Principle 8. *Do Not Eat Just Before Going to Sleep*

The greatest period of physical healing occurs during sleep. This is the time the body does housekeeping by moving wastes from the cellular level to the main excretory functions. If the stomach is still digesting food during this time, the body must divert energy to digestion and away from necessary maintenance.

An overfilled stomach presses against the liver, restricting its work of detoxification and hampering the processing of food in the small intestine. The bile it produces cannot get to the small intestine as well, collects in the gallbladder and liver, and thereby forms stones. Remember, the stomach is most active in the morning; then its activity slows down. During the day there is more energy in the small intestine, and during the night the liver does its important work of detoxification.

A person who eats before sleep poisons his or her body, and feels more tired in the morning than before sleep. Small wonder, since all night long his or her body worked and choked from the internal pressure and toxicity.

The distribution of meals across the span of the day should be in sync with the body's biorhythms, a person's individual characteristics, and his or her work schedule.

The last meal must be no later than a minimum of at least 3-4 hours before sleep.

Most people eat three times a day, however, depending on what you eat, you can eat 2, 3, or 4 times a day.

If your food consists of fruits and juices that are quickly digested, you may eat every 2-4 hours. For vegetables, grains, nuts, fish, and meat, the time between meals should be 4-7 hours and more. Under these conditions you should not eat more than 2-3 times per day. For some people with slow digestion, once a day is enough.

14

Principle 9. *Do Not Eat Unless Hungry*

People often complain about bad digestion; however, it is we ourselves who make the choices that can decrease or increase bad digestion.

When you eat not because you're hungry but because of some other reason such as it is time for dinner or due to social or recreational reasons, etc., your digestion will be poor. When we eat without hunger, the digestive organs are not ready for the work so there aren't enough digestive juices available. Further, the body may be solving other serious problems, such as digesting the previous meal, fighting off an infection, neutralizing toxins, etc.

Digestion is most efficient when you feel hunger. If you wait for strong hunger before eating, the results go beyond good digestion. **A hungry stomach produces very acidic peptic juice, which destroys harmful bacteria, neutralizes toxins and cleanses the blood.** Of course, such "miracles" only happen if you follow all other principles as well.

There is also a very simple way to improve the action of your digestive juices. Ten to 30 minutes after you eat, put a pinch of sea salt on the tip of your tongue. Wait for the salt to dissolve and swallow the saliva.

Principle 10. *Choose Food That Brings You Health*

We usually eat to satisfy our mind or curiosity or to quench discomfort in the stomach. The primary goal of eating, the goal of giving vital nutrition to organs and cells, is too often forgotten.

Naturally, the nutrition that our organs and cells desire and the food that our mind and tongue want can be sharply different. We need to realize that not everything which is tasty on the tongue will be good for the system. It is important to remember that the food we eat becomes part of our bodies, our cells and organs. Our health depends on the health of our inner organs, and the health of our inner organs depends on the quality of our food.

If a house is built with inferior brick and cement, it will not withstand strong wind and other destructive forces. It is the same with our organs. If they are built with healthy food, they will withstand the tests that life will throw at them: cold, heat, stresses, work overloads, etc. When choosing the right food to eat, you should take into account not only general recommendations from books on diet, from Aurveda, and from blood type books, but also your personal traits that only you can know. **Choosing food that brings you health means also avoiding food that does not agree with your system.**

Ask yourself this critical question: "Do you live to eat, or do you eat to live?" The answer you give to this simple question will determine many of your life and health issues.

Principle 11. *Eat Food According to Season*

Food is imported to America from all over the globe, so in our grocery stores there are no "seasonal" products. However, seasonality does matter for the human body. Fruits and berries are warm-season foods and cool the body; they are balanced by the hot weather. In the winter, such cooling can lead to weakness and disease.

In the winter you should eat food that increases body temperature: slightly stewed vegetables, grains, nuts, hot pepper, onion, summer-and-winter radish (Raphanus sativus), garlic, ginger, butter, fish etc.

16

Of course, neither in summer nor in winter can you completely avoid the mixing of food, but seasonal products should dominate.

Principle 12. *Eat Food Grown in Your Area*

This principle is more do-able for owners of farms and gardens. The point of this advice is that all life adapts to the conditions in which it lives, whether that life is human, plant or animal. When this principle is followed, the food creates balance and harmony in the organism.

Principle 13. *Do Not Eat under Stress*

Some people lose their appetite when stressed, but most eat non-stop when they are nervous.

When you are stressed, your food is saturated with the vibrations of the emotion that you are experiencing, and the negative energy of the emotion remains in your body for a long time. The digestive organs themselves turn off completely under stress because all the energy of the body is routed to the brain and muscles.

Such eating will only cause harm. Why then do people eat under stress? Because the food distracts them from the problem temporarily, and they find calmness in that distraction.

There are other, healthier ways to re-orient the body during stress. The purpose of these methods is to distract the body from one problem and attract it to another, harmless or even desirable problem. The method described in this book is also medicative. See Book 3, the chapter on cleansing from negative emotions.

Principle 14. *While Eating, Do Not Talk about Serious or Disturbing Topics*

This includes discussing the behavior of your spouse or children, watching television, etc. During your meals, your attention should be focused on the process of chewing and on the taste of the food. Think about how the best of this food will be assimilated by your body and will make it stronger. Think about how the unnecessary components of this food will be easily and promptly eliminated. As it is well known, the thoughts that dominate in your mind are the ones that form your life. **Learn to govern your thoughts, and your life and health will improve.**

Principle 15. *Do Not Eat When Seriously Ill*

During acute disease, such as high fever, flu, sharp pain in the digestive tract, or nausea, etc., all the body's energy is absorbed in fighting the problem. Appetite is usually absent at such times, and it would be wrong to force food into the stomach, artificially attracting to the stomach the body energy that is so needed for other, bigger, vital problems.

During nausea, cold, cough, and other problems, you should first cleanse the stomach and the large intestine and then, when your condition improves, drink calming herbal extracts and fresh juices. Only when true hunger appears should you begin to eat, and that carefully.

Principle 16. *How to Activate Digestion*

For better assimilation of nutrients from food, it is important to help organs start actively digesting. There are some rather simple methods that can be used after finishing the meal. Close the left nostril with a piece of cotton and breathe for 10-15 minutes a bit deeper than usual through the right nostril. Breathing through the right nostril heats the body; breathing through the left nostril cools the body. It is precisely internal warmth that activates digestion.

Take a light walk outdoors for 15-20 minutes. Massage your stomach clockwise this whole time. The walk will slightly deepen your breathing and will give your body oxygen that is necessary for good digestion. The light massage will improve circulation in the digestive organs, activate the secretion of digestive juices, and help remove the blockages created by gasses and refuse in the digestive tract. If you have good digestion, you should feel the desire to use the bathroom after the walk.

Some other suggestions from Aurveda to improve digestion:
• Drink hot, fresh ginger tea.
• Eat warm food, and add some spices like chile peppers or curries.
• Eat foods which have a bitter taste (salads, spinach, kale)
• Eat a ginger pickle before lunch or dinner to increase your "digestive fire."

To make a ginger pickle, sprinkle lemon juice and a pinch of sea salt on a thin slice of fresh ginger. Eat this ginger pickle 15 minutes before a meal.

• Take 2-3 sips of hot water every 10-15 minutes during the day. This is also good to prevent and treat colds and sore throat.

• 30-60 minutes after a meal take a pinch of sea salt on your tongue, and after the salt is dissolved, swallow the saliva and spit out any remaining salt crystals.

Principle 17. *Do Not Eat Very Cold Food*

The process of digesting food in the stomach begins only when the food we have eaten reaches body temperature. Therefore, cold foods must be heated by the body and hot foods must be cooled by the body before proper digestion can begin. When you eat room-temperature food, say 68-73° F, your body spends energy to heat it to the required 97-98° F, a difference of 25-34° F.

If you chew your food thoroughly it will be heated significantly while still in the mouth. By chewing well, you will save a lot of digestive energy and shorten the time before digestion begins.

But if you eat very cold food (below about 40° F), or drink cold fluids with ice, or have ice cream for dessert, you chill not only the stomach, but also all nearby digestive organs. To start digesting the consumed food, the stomach needs to heat it from 40° F to 98° F, a difference of 58° F. Especially if you ate a lot, this may take hours of pointless waste of digestive energy. When the temperature of the food eaten finally reaches the temperature of the stomach, there will be very little energy left for digestion itself. Digestion will be poor and will give the body more toxins than nutrients.

Ideally, the temperature of the prepared food should be the same as or a little above the temperature of the body. After refrigeration, raw, fresh food should stay for awhile at room temperature to warm up. Food at room temperature should be thoroughly chewed to begin warming to body temperature.

The same principles apply to all drinks. If you like cold drinks, one piece of ice added will help to give drinks at room temperature enough of the cool taste you are looking for. Then the cooled drink can be held in the mouth not only to mix with saliva, which is very important, but also to begin heating. After all, it is easier to heat a small gulp in the mouth than a large amount of liquid in the stomach.

Principle 18. *Let Your Digestive Tract Rest*

The digestive organs work for years and decades without any rest other than the hours of sleep. They rarely get a real vacation. The modern person, nurtured by pharmaceuticals and raised on the couch in front of the television, comes to believe that he or she must eat incessantly to survive, or to remain strong. This is reinforced by advertisements on television and in magazines that are strictly designed to make you want to eat their food.

Except for those organs (like the heart) that are designed to work non-stop, no organ should be worked continuously when it indeed can be rested. Just as sleep for the body is as natural as eating to live, so also rest for the organs is natural and beneficial. Overworked organs (such as the colon and the stomach) can be weakened by relentlessly driving them, and this can sabotage the entire body.

All religions in the world have one thing in common; they all recommend regular fasting. Regular fasting "unloads" the digestive system and makes a person closer to nature and to God.

21

Depending on your weight and health, you may conduct "unloading days" of 24-36 hours once every 1-2 weeks. You can choose among these different types of unloading diet:

- Drink only fresh juices of fruits and vegetables.
- Drink vegetable decoctions.
- Drink herbal extracts.
- Drink only water.
- Eat and drink nothing.
- Eat only easily digestible fruits and berries: watermelon, other melons, peaches, grapes, most berries, etc.

Principle 19. *Regularly Cleanse Your Digestive Organs*

No one ever had to tell you that if you eat something rotten it is bad for you. We are naturally repelled by spoiled foods, and naturally drawn to properly ripened foods. This is good since spoiled foods have extra toxins in them.

Most people understand that toxins may enter the body through air, food, and drink; through the skin; or via drugs. But not everyone understands that even **the best organic food also creates some refuse or waste in the body.** All human activities create waste: the building of a house, cooking, sewing, breathing, etc. Chewing leaves a yellow residue on the teeth. The process of digestion leaves a layer of residue on the sides of the stomach.

The activity of each organ and each cell of the body produces wastes that must be eliminated. Every organ and every cell not only consumes nutrients, but also has a cleansing function to eliminate the wastes generated in burning or digesting that nutrition.

However, not all of these wastes created by digestion or brought in from outside the body can be readily eliminated.

Slowly but surely, the amount of toxins from these wastes builds up. These toxins poison and weaken the entire body. To rid the body of collected waste and keep it clean, we need to knowledgeably and consciously help the body cleanse itself. Periodically it is necessary to conduct a general cleanup of the body, that is, a deep internal cleansing of the organs. For complete details of this process see my book, *Deep Internal Body Cleansing*.

If you realize the importance of cleansing the body, and if you include this cleansing in your life's schedule, you will receive the key to preventing and curing many diseases.

"Now I Have Lots of Energy"

When I came to Dr. Koyfman last year, I was not doing very well with my diet and had a lack of energy. My gall bladder was giving me terrible problems. The only other option would have been to have it removed. My mother told me that was out of the question. She had been going to Dr. Koyfman for awhile and told me she was taking me to him.

I went through the colon, small intestine, liver, stomach, lymph, and cell cleanses, which included a seven-day fast. I have never felt better. This helped me to improve my diet and exercise on a daily basis, and now I have lots of energy to do things I could never do. I would like to thank Dr. Koyfman and my mother for helping me get to this great health I have today.

I still have my gall bladder and my system is working extremely well. Thank you very much.

—Suzanne Slaton

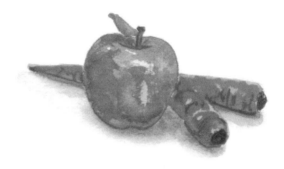

Other Principles and Components of Healthy Digestion

Methods of Consuming Air

While we can live without food for a month or more, and without water for several days, we will last only several minutes without air. Thus, **air is the most important nutrient.**

It is precisely this important source of nutrition and life that we think about least. The air in the buildings where we spend most of our time is absolutely unpalatable. Usually there are unventilated, or poorly ventilated, rooms or cubicles whose air contains unhealthful additions from the heater or the air conditioner and used-up air from human lungs. This air can also contain cigarette smoke and other poisons.

The air outdoors, on busy streets, contains plenty of unhealthful additions in the form of toxins and heavy metals

24

from vehicle exhaust. Near airports the air can be so bad that it can damage the paint on cars parked at the airport.

Even if you regularly ventilate your room or find a park where the air is cleaner, that is not enough. **To make sure that oxygen gets to all of your body's cells,** to make sure that it aids in the digestive and oxygenation processes, you should **open up your lungs** and activate your circulation.

The methodology of opening the lungs includes fast walking or light running and breathing exercises according to the systems of yoga and tai-chi. Some exercises are described in the chapter on lung cleansing in my Book 1. More detailed descriptions of these breathing techniques can be found in books on yoga and tai-chi.

Now we come to a very important conclusion: **If the main ingredients of nutrition—air, water, and food—are high-quality and correctly consumed, they not only feed the body but also cleanse it.**

The converse is also true: **Cleansing the body, especially its digestive organs—the small and large intestines, the liver, the stomach, and the pancreas—improves its nutrition.** To improve the body is to improve its nutrition and strengthen its immunity and health.

Caution: It is very important to learn how to breathe correctly under professional guidance because **incorrect breathing can lead to disease.** Deep and frequent breathing without physical activity flushes carbon dioxide from the system, constricts the blood vessels, and restricts the distribution of oxygen. Deep breathing without physical activity becomes beneficial only when it is slow and has pauses between inhalation and exhalation as done in Yoga or Tai Chi. When we are not active, correct breathing is shallow without deep inhalation and exhalation. We can slow the inhalations and exhalations with conscious relaxation of our muscles. The more the muscles relax, the more shallow becomes our breathing. This creates more carbon dioxide in the system which expands the blood vessels and allows more oxygen to be absorbed. This is only the briefest information on right breathing. To learn correct breathing, you need to find a professional guide.

Methods of Consuming Water

Two thirds of the human body is water. Water is the primary ingredient in the formation of blood, lymph, saliva, gastric juice, tissue fluids, etc. Drinking water thins the blood, which eases the work of the heart. If we do not drink enough water, the blood becomes viscous and difficult for the heart to pump through the veins, arteries, and especially the capillaries. In this case we feel exhausted, because a tired heart makes the whole body tired.

The water in the blood is the main carrier for transporting nutrients and oxygen to the cells. Water dilutes the body's toxins and helps them to be washed out through urine, sweat, and intestines.

To aid the body in cleansing itself, you need to drink one or two large glasses of clean water three times daily. A good time to do this is upon rising and 15-30 minutes before each meal. Do not drink water during meals. Wait 1-2 hours after the meal before drinking again and then do it only by sipping a little at a time. It is also best to quit drinking an hour before sleep. At that time you may drink ½-1 glass of calming tea.

From this you can see that **water is a very important nutrient in the human diet. Its amount and quality play an important role in sustaining health.**

Before continuing to the description of living food, I want to make a short stop on one more very important nutrient.

How Many Times per Day Is it Necessary to Eat?

Wild nature has a lot of variety. Birds nibble grain and catch insects all day. Predators often measure their time between meals in days. There are animals that eat once per week or even once per year. A lot depends on the speed of metabolism.

People also vary in how often they eat. Some eat 5-6 times per day, others 2-3 times. Some eat once a day, although in that one time they try to eat everything that they did not eat during the day.

So how many times do you need to eat to be healthy? It is recommended to feed an infant every 4-5 hours. An adult needs as much or more time between meals, depending on the amount and type of food consumed. The time to digest fruit is 2-4 hours. Sour fruits are digested faster, sweet ones slower. Vegetables require 3-5 hours, grain needs 4-5 hours, nuts and seeds take 4-6 hours. Food combinations prolong the digestion time. Eating only one type of product speeds up digestion. Also, digestion time is affected by age, the health of the digestive tract, whether you chew well, whether you felt hunger, the time of the day, the amount of food, the presence of stress, physical activity, etc.

That is why it's impossible to name a precise amount of time needed for digestion. For different people and for each specific situation, the time will be different.

It is also worth noting that what is meant here is not the time that food needs to pass through the whole digestive tract, but only the time required to pass through the stomach. If we discuss the complete absorption of nutrients, this process begins in the mouth and continues in the stomach. Then most of the nutrients are absorbed in the small intestine, and a bit more in the large intestine. Therefore, the "time of digestion" that we discuss here is the time food spends in the stomach.

Although we may feel hunger when food leaves the stomach, the body continues to receive nutrients from the food in the small intestine. In fact, this is where the greatest amount of nutrients is absorbed. The hunger does not mean that the body is short of nutrients.

Instead, in prehistoric times this sensation told humans to start looking for food. This could take hours or even days. While the person searched for food with such difficulty, the previous meal continued to supply the body with nutrients. Before the previous meal was finished, something that can take 5-12 hours, our ancestors found new food. We moderns, on the other hand, get scared of the sense of hunger and hurry to put something in our mouth, afraid that if we don't, we will weaken or starve to death. This fear is unfounded. **Skipped meals allow the body to conserve digestive energy, which it uses to cleanse and defend itself.** This means that **conserving digestive energy increases immunity.** That is why I recommend eating two meals, and for some people one meal, per day.

This arrangement of the diet lets you receive more nutrients and less waste, resulting in less toxicity. Such a diet also lets you receive more energy for work, exercise, and other activities. That is, **if you do not overload your body with digesting food that it doesn't need, your overall health improves.**

What should you do at times when you skip meals? Drink! Drink one or two cups of fresh juice, herbal tea, or just water.

Main Foods To Eat

- Wild greens, if you are knowledgeable about them.
- Sprouts.
- Fruits, vegetables, and their juices.
- Green leafy vegetables.
- Seeds and nuts.
- Cold pressed vegetable oil and ghee.
- Whole grain, sprouting grain.

- Fresh fish from uncontaminated waters
- Organic meat.

It depends on the specific person whether that person should eat meat, be a vegetarian, or eat only raw food. It is more important here whether you follow dietary principles than whether you eat meat or not. If you account for the kind of meat that it is, how it should be prepared, how it combines with other foods, etc., and if your body can digest it, there will be no serious problems.

My preference is with vegetarianism, in which you eat 80% raw food and 20% fresh prepared food. I also recommend 2-4 periods per year, lasting 2-4 weeks, when you eat only raw food. **This dietary system will do a good job of supplying your body with living products, and will not cut you off from society and the real conditions of modern life.**

It is easiest to conduct a program of "raw foods only" during the summer, when many fruits, berries, and vegetables are in season. This program can also include raw fresh juices for the purpose of cleansing the body while feeding it. Of course, for the body to be cleansed completely, you need to give it extra help. See the chapter on cell cleansing in my book, *Deep Internal Body Cleansing.*

Wild Greens

If you were to analyze the diet of centenarians (people who live to be 100 years old or older), you would find that most of them consumed **wild** greens. Wild greens have a certain vital potential. While domestic plants need constant care and irrigation to make them grow and prevent them from dying, wild plants grow successfully without any care. Moreover, they grow even if you cut them down or trample on them. That's how much life force they have.

If you had a large enough collection of edible wild greens, their dietary value would probably be enough to make food supplements completely unnecessary. However, to eat edible wild greens that can be found in a park, a forest, or even in your back yard, you need to be educated by a knowledgeable person. Otherwise you may make a mistake and eat something harmful. Additionally, plants found in parks may be contaminated with any number of chemicals.

Sprouts

Sprouts change the dormant energy of grain into the energy of motion, growth, and life. The time of sprouting is the most robust time of the plant. Although the sprout does not contain all the nutrients that the future fruit will, it contains the program of development and growth of the plant. Most likely, it also contains growth hormones and substances that defend the plant against parasites. This makes sprouts a great food for the endocrine and immune systems.

Many books explain the methodology of growing sprouts in your own kitchen. My favorite is a book by Steve Meyerovitz, entitled, *Sprout It.*

Supplements

Supplements are what we use to supply the nutrients that are missing in our food.

Intensive methods of cultivating the soil and growing food have robbed the soil of its minerals. The soil no longer contains enough minerals for plants to grow, as was made clear in a 1936 United States Senate document describing the poorness of American soil. It stated that 70 minerals and other elements are necessary for healthy, nutritious food crops. According to this government report, American soil no longer naturally had these 70 elements, and farmers were only replacing the three necessary for healthy looking plants.

Often plants don't receive even the minerals that are still left in the soil because they are harvested before they ripen, in order to increase their shelf life. As a result, plants don't receive enough of either minerals or solar energy. When we eat such products, we do not receive enough nutrients as in vitamins, minerals and enzymes.

On the other hand, the body that is filled with toxins attracts parasites, which find excellent conditions for their growth and proliferation in such a toxic environment. Born in the filth, the parasite steals from its host important nutrients, minerals, hormones, etc., from the host's blood and tissue, and from the food eaten by the host.

31

As a result, a deficit of nutrients appears in the body. The shortage of nutrients can lead to serious diseases and disorders. To avoid this, it is necessary to take food supplements. In order to supply your body with enough supplements, feed the armies of parasites, and replace the nutrients kept from the bloodstream by the thick layer of toxins on the sides of the intestines, you would have to take "tons" of vitamin and mineral supplements. However, if you cleanse your body of parasites and toxins, you will need to feed only yourself and you can do that much more efficiently. In that case, you will need a much smaller amount of supplements.

In any case, you must remember: **supplements are useful only if you follow the main principles of proper eating. Otherwise, their usefulness is negligible.** To determine which supplements you need, it is best to consult with a specialist who can take into account your health goals.

The Importance of Kitchen Equipment

Just as it is hard to go anywhere in a big city without a car, so it is also difficult to improve your diet and keep it healthy without quality kitchen equipment. Good kitchen equipment eases and speeds up the preparation of food, **improves its taste and appearance, and facilitates the absorption of nutrients.**

Juicer

Fresh juices are biologically active fluids that contain vitamins, minerals, and enzymes in a living state. They have healing properties. They are easily and quickly digested, have a pleasant taste, quickly satiate you, and give you energy. The digestion of freshly extracted juice takes only 15-30 minutes, thereby conserving digestive energy. **This energy is freed for use by the immune system.** In other words, **drinking juices increases your immunity to disease.** Fresh juices also cleanse and rejuvenate the organism and normalize body weight. Cheap juicers can't extract all nutrients. A lot of nutrients remain in the pulp and are thrown away with the pulp. Some high-quality juicers are made by Green Rower, Green Life, and Norwalk. These juicers extract the greatest amount of nutrients. Each of them has its advantages, but the most affordable and practical one is made by Champion for commercial use. You can even use it to prepare a healthy fruit and nut ice cream.

Blender

The blender turns whole products into liquid. This liquid contains both pulp and fresh biological juice. A good blender pulverizes food so much that it is easier to digest. For example, a lot of people cannot eat nuts and sunflower seeds, which are good sources of protein. These foods give them gas and blockages. However, if the nuts are mixed with a juice and processed in a blender, the gas problem disappears.

Thus, foods prepared in a blender, like fresh juices, can contain enzymes, vitamins, and minerals. They can also contain fats, proteins, and carbohydrates.

A blender can be used to make smoothies, protein shakes, raw soups, dressings, gravies, etc. You can also use it to make very good wheat grass juice. The best blender is made by Vita-Mix.

Food Processor

Raw salads from vegetables and fruits are the chief part of a healthy diet. Vegetables and fruits processed in a food processor look more appetizing. They are easier to chew and contain more juice. There are both manual and electric food processors. The most recommended models are made by Cuisinart.

Dehydrator

Useful for heating and drying fruit and vegetable chips, and products made of grain, nuts, and seeds. The main characteristic of a good dehydrator is that its temperature should not rise higher than 105°. Higher temperatures destroy enzymes.

Meat Grinder

In a healthy diet the meat grinder is used for grinding nuts, seeds, and dried fruits, as well as for grinding sprouting grain to make healthy bread, etc. For a recipe for bread made from sprouting wheat, read my book, *Unique Method of Colon Rejuvenation.*

A meat grinder can also be used to make *healthy* candy, cakes, etc.

Many books on diet include descriptions of additional kinds of kitchen equipment. If you are curious about your health, you should constantly read, watching for novelties, because our world is ever-changing. New and useful knowledge gives us the interest and energy to live.

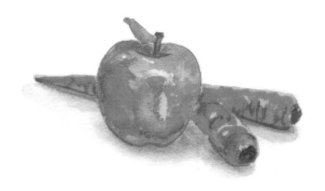

Recipes for Living Food

The Best Way to Preserve Nutrients

In unprocessed food products the most important components are enzymes, vitamins, minerals, carbohydrates, etc., in their natural, living state. Various ways of processing raw products, by dicing, shredding, grinding, etc., reduce their biological value, especially if food is preserved for a while after processing.

On the other hand, we are accustomed to food processed by cooking, roasting, baking, etc., and to its taste and appearance. The transition from the usual diet becomes easier when the new dishes are similar in taste and appearance to the dishes we usually eat.

Preparing such dishes takes time and planning, i.e., soaking, sprouting, etc., yet in the real, practical conditions of the life of working people who are used to eating canned or restaurant food instead of cooking, these expenditures of time might seem too much.

Here is a solution. Those who have the time and desire to prepare complicated recipes can use recipes from the many books on living food. For those who do not have that kind of time, I will try to provide simple recipes that take no more, and often less, than twenty minutes to prepare. If you want to use sprouts, you can buy them in health stores or learn to make them yourself.

If you want to get more nutrients, remember, **the simpler a recipe is, the more valuable it is.**

When using a recipe, seek to understand the principles involved. Then later on, you can also think up your own recipes, and when you begin to create, a genuine interest in what you are doing naturally develops.

The First Chinese Wisdom

Eat a hearty breakfast. In the East the saying is to eat your own breakfast without sharing it, then for lunch share some of your food with your friends, and for supper give your meal to your enemy. In the West there is a similar saying that advises you to eat like a king for breakfast, eat like a merchant for lunch, and eat like a pauper in the evening.

The meaning here is to eat a big breakfast to carry you through the day, eat a moderate meal at midday that won't slow you down, and in the evening eat a small meal.

According to Oriental tradition, breakfast must be nutritious and whole. What can be more nutritious than fresh juices of fruits, vegetables, nuts, and berries in their raw form? These products contain a large amount of nutrients, are easy to digest, and help to cleanse the body. The recipes given here for breakfast sufficiently satisfy these conditions. With the phrase, "whole and nutritious diet," Oriental wisdom means not huge amounts of food dumped in the stomach and impossible to digest, but easily digestible products that saturate the blood with nutrients.

Breakfast Options

1. Fresh Orange Juice

See recipe 2 for preparation instructions.

2. Juice Made of Two Oranges and One Grapefruit

Preparation instructions: Wash the grapefruit and oranges. Remove the rind (yellow or orange outer skin) but leave the white inner part. Cut into segments and juice them in your Champion juicer. Repeat this three to five times, until the pulp becomes sufficiently dry. Drink 1-3 cups of juice per day. Chew your juices as if they were a solid food.

3. Fruit Cocktail

Ingredients: 1 banana, 1 cup seedless grapes, 3-4 ice cubes made of filtered water.

Preparation instructions: Peel the banana and break it into small pieces. Wash the grapes, separate them from the branches and dry them in air or with a paper towel. Put all ingredients into the Vita-Mix and blend at high speed for 20-30 seconds. **Variations:** You can replace the grapes with a pineapple or an orange, and the banana with mango or papaya.

4. Protein Shake

Ingredients: 1 grapefruit, 2 oranges, a handful of cashew or macadamia nuts, 1 tablespoon of fresh or frozen cranberries, 1 teaspoon of wild greens from Nature's First Food, 1 teaspoon of papazime (an enzyme which helps to digest protein), 3-4 ice cubes.

Preparation instructions: Wash the grapefruit and oranges. Remove the rind (yellow or orange outer skin) but leave the white inner part. Juice the grapefruit and the oranges in the Champion juicer. Pour this juice into the Vita-Mix. Drop in all other ingredients and turn the mixer on at high speed. Let it work for one minute. The ice cubes prevent the juice from overheating and help preserve the enzymes; they also improve the taste of the beverage.

Note: It is not recommended that you drink such a beverage more than 3 times per week. Two or three times per week is perfectly enough.

5. Melon

A melon can make a superb breakfast. You can eat it as it is, as a juice, or pulverized in the blender.

Note: Do not be afraid of eating a melon if you have yeast problems. Melon is a great anti-parasitic food, and has effective cleansing properties.

6. Watermelon

As with any melon, watermelon can be blended, juiced or eaten solid, but eat enough to be satisfied.

7. Any Fruits and Berries Your Body Accepts

It is important to note that, if you have yeast infection, it is better to eat sour fruit. If you sometimes want to eat sweet fruit, eat it with warm herbal tea. The tea "Calli" has a very good taste. By drinking tea with sweet fruit, you reduce the concentration of sugar, i.e., you won't feed the yeast.

8. Green Juices

Juices made from cucumber, celery, romaine lettuce, kale, etc., can be consumed at breakfast. They can also be mixed with pineapple, apple or carrot juice for taste, in a 60/40 proportion, 60% of green and 40% of sweet or sour-sweet juices.

Examples of green juices:
- 4 celery ribs + ½ head of cabbage.
- 4 celery ribs + ½ cucumber + ½ cup parsley.
- 4 celery ribs + 1 cup of dandelion ribs.
- 4-5 celery ribs + ½ head of lettuce + ½ cup of spinach.

9. Energy Cocktail

If you have physically demanding work or exercises to do, add 1-2 tablespoons of cold pressed flax seed oil to your juice. The natural fat in the cold pressed oil is an excellent source of energy. Taken with the juice, it will retard the absorption of vitamins, minerals, etc., into the blood. The fat and nutrients will enter the blood in small portions and supply the working muscles with energy.

The juice with 1-2 tablespoons of cold pressed oil will not overload the digestive system, and the absorption of the nutrients into the blood will be akin to sprinkling.

You can pour a barrel of water under a tree, but its roots will not be able to absorb it all at once. The excess will simply sink into the ground or evaporate. After awhile the tree will become short of water again.

Sprinkling is completely different. When water gets to the roots slowly they can absorb all of it. While in the first case most of the water was lost, in the second 100% of it is used by the tree over a long time, during which the tree feeds its trunk, branches, leaves, and fruit.

If we drink a lot of juice at once, it is quickly absorbed. The cells cannot use all of the nutrients at once, and excess fluid will be excreted through the kidneys, carrying most of the nutrients with it. There is nothing wrong with that, because with the excess fluid the kidneys excrete waste materials; however, it is much more less trouble and less expensive to do that with water rather than with juice.

When we want to efficiently use the nutrients in fresh juice in order to perform hard work or exercise, it is best to add cold pressed flax seed oil or cold pressed olive oil to the juice. **In this case we lose not a single gram of nutrient, receive a lot of energy, and feel no hunger for a long time.** Besides having great energy value, such a drink helps cleanse the intestines, since the cold pressed oil has laxative properties.

Thus, juice mixed with cold pressed oil uses nutrients efficiently, gives you energy, and cleanses the body. Nuts and avocado mixed with juice in a blender have the same effect.

40

Another way to not lose the nutrients in fresh juice is to drink it in small gulps, holding each gulp in your mouth for 10-20 seconds.

10. A Bigger Breakfast

The recipes provided above work best for individuals who feel not very hungry but more physically active in the morning. Those who feel more hungry in the morning would be hard to satisfy with juice or a smoothie. For these individuals I can recommend the following breakfast. This type of food might seem strange to eat for breakfast; however, it will leave the body satisfied and balanced for the whole day.

Option #1
- Fresh, raw salad *(see page 45)*.
- Porridge (whole grains only). *See instructions on page 59.*

Option #2
- A glass of fresh vegetable juice
- Porridge with slightly cooked vegetables

Look for recipes in Lunch and Supper sections which follow.

When choosing your perfect breakfast, it is very important to follow some main rules. Always start your meals with raw salad or at least a piece of any raw vegetable. You may also start with a glass of fresh vegetable juice. Only then, you may eat freshly cooked foods. By following these rules and considering proper food combining, you can make up your own recipes according to your individual taste and preference.

The Second Chinese Wisdom

Share your lunch with a friend. Remember, before food gives your body nutrients and energy, it consumes energy from the body for the work of digestion. So, if you eat harsh or incompatible food or overload the body with a large volume of food, such a lunch would make you want to sleep, not work.

Aurveda, the science about how to live long and be healthy, says that between 12 and 3 p.m. the sun is straight overhead and radiates the greatest amount of heat. Since heat is a required condition for good digestion, many authorities think that the largest meal should be eaten at this time.

Chinese folk medicine claims that the greatest activity during the three hours after noon occurs in the small intestine, and that the stomach is most active in the morning, about 7-9 a.m.

Putting these two ideas together, if in the morning you eat fruits or nut milk, the food will reach the small intestine at precisely the best time for intestinal digestion, and the digestion and absorption of nutrients at this time will be greatest. So the digestion of the previous meal will be most efficient, but not so with the new meal. The digestion of food that is eaten during lunch comes at a time when digestive energy in the stomach has waned somewhat. Thus, it is wrong to gorge yourself at this time.

This then is the wisdom behind the famous Chinese saying: **"Eat breakfast yourself, share your lunch with a friend, and give your supper to your enemy."**

So how should we eat during lunch to satisfy hunger and at the same time conserve energy?

- Eat small amounts of food. While you can load your stomach to 2/3 of its volume at breakfast, at lunch you should eat a little less than approximately 50% of stomach volume. How to calculate the volume of your stomach was explained earlier.

- Eat simple food: salads, soups, etc.
- It is better to eat raw food, although it's permissible to add some cooked food, especially in the winter.
- The number of ingredients shouldn't be greater than 5-7, or, even better, 3-5.
- Food must not form a large amount of gas. If raw food forms gas, then it contains a large amount of chemical additives. Even if the label says "organic," that guarantees nothing. In this case, use digestive enzymes. If enzymes don't help, exclude this product from your diet.

To satisfy your hunger and feel the taste of food, you must pay attention to the chewing process. Details are in the chapter on "Koyfman Fasting©" in my book, *Deep Internal Body Cleansing*.

Lunch

The average person has lunch at work five or six times a week. Of course, there is no time to actually prepare during lunch break, so most people eat at various fast food restaurants where the cooking hygiene, technology, and food quality are all questionable.

Certainly you can find good places to eat, usually health restaurants, juice bars, etc. However, if you are serious about your health, **nobody can prepare your food better than you**. Prepare the food yourself, or let a relative or close friend do it for you. Simple food prepared with care and positive thoughts is best for your health.

So when should you prepare food, if there is no time at work?

Most of the preparations should be made beforehand, preferably in the evening. Part of the job can be done in the morning. All you have to do at work is to add the dressing, which can also be made beforehand.

Some Simple Lunch Recipes

For people who prefer to eat raw food, **raw salads are the main part of the diet.** It is best to make the salads from vegetables currently in season. The more nutritious salads are made from the **roots, leaves, and fruits** of the plants. For preparation, a food processor is best, although a good knife can be used instead.

As you remember, if you eating away from home, you should make preparations in the evening. But if you have the opportunity to do this right before the meal, nothing can be better. Freshly prepared food has a higher energy and nutritive value. However, let us account for real conditions and do what is most appropriate at the time.

1. Salad from White Cabbage, Carrot, and Onion

Wash 2-3 carrots, cut off both ends. Chose and clean half as much cabbage as carrot, and one half of an onion. Put the carrot through a food processor; cabbage and onion can be diced with a knife. Mix everything and place it in a closed container in the refrigerator. It would also be nice to add a pinch of finely diced dill to such a salad.

44

Dressing: 1 Tbs. lemon juice, 1-2 Tbs. cold pressed olive oil, 1 Tbs. Nama Shoyu. Mix the ingredients and then pour the dressing into a small glass bottle with a hermetical stopper and put it in the refrigerator. Mix dressing with salad immediately before the meal.

With the salad it is permissible to eat 5-10 olives. Soak them in pure water for an hour or two if they have a lot of salt or vinegar in them. However, it is best to eat quality olives.

2. Salad from Tomatoes, Cucumbers, Onions, Parsley Tops, and Sunflower Sprouts

If these products are washed and the cucumbers cleaned previously, it is quite easy to dice them with a knife immediately before the meal. The dressing is the same as in recipe #1.

This salad can be sprinkled with ground sunflower seeds, flax seeds or walnuts. These raw seeds or nuts may have mold or fungi on them that you do not want. To fix this simple problem, heat them in the oven or on the stove top for 1-2 minutes. This will kill the mold and fungi without harming the seeds or nuts. Once this is done, give them a twirl in a blender. It is better to store the resulting powder, not in a refrigerator, but in a freezer, in a closed bottle, with sea salt added. The proportion of salt to food powder should be 1:10.

3. Salad from Marinated Greens

Ingredients: 1 bunch romaine lettuce, 1 bunch kale, ½ cup grated carrots, ½ cup grated zucchini.

Simple Marinade: 2 lemons, juiced, ½ cup cold pressed olive oil, ¼ cup Nama Shoyu or sea salt for taste.

Wash the kale greens and cut out the stems. Wash the romaine lettuce. Cut kale and romaine lettuce into small pieces. Mix all vegetables with marinade and toss until well coated. Cover the greens, vegetables and marinade in the refrigerator overnight.

4. Salad from Fresh Roots

Ingredients: 4-5 carrots, 1-2 celery roots, 2-3 Jerusalem artichokes, 2 oz. apple juice from your juicer, 1 oz. cold pressed olive oil.

Grate in food processor the carrots, celery root, and artichokes. Mix apple juice with cold pressed olive oil and pour over the salad.

5. Salad from Cabbage, Carrots, and Sunflower Seeds

Ingredients: 1/3 medium-sized cabbage, 4-5 carrots, 1 oz. sunflower seeds, 1 Tbs. cold pressed olive oil, 1 tsp. mustard, 1 tsp. honey.

Cut cabbage into small pieces, grate carrots, and mix together. Sprinkle with sunflower seeds. Mix cold pressed olive oil, mustard, and honey, and pour over the salad.

6. Salad from Carrots, Beets (Cooked or Raw), Nuts, and Garlic

Ingredients: 3-4 carrots, 1 beet root, 4-5 Tbs. walnuts, 2-3 cloves garlic, 2 Tbs. cold pressed olive oil or cold pressed flax seed oil.

Grate the carrots in a food processor. Use the blade to process the beet, nuts, and garlic. Mix with grated carrots and cold pressed olive oil.

This salad is very nutritious. It helps to create red blood cells and is good for those who have anemia.

7. Salad from Cauliflower

Ingredients: 2 cups cauliflower, 2 ½ cups water, 2-3 basil leaves, 2-3 black peppercorns, 1 lemon juiced, 1 tsp. honey, garnish or parsley and dill greens.

Prepare the cauliflower by cutting thin stems into small pieces, peeling thick stems and cutting them into small pieces, including the leaves whole, and setting aside the flower. Put stems and leaves in water with basil leaves and black peppercorns and cook to make a broth. Cool the broth and add to it the lemon juice and honey. Then cut the flower of the cauliflower into small pieces and pour the broth over it.

This salad has a good taste, activates digestion, and helps to cleanse the kidneys and liver.

8. Dressings

Dressings help to improve the taste of the salads besides making them more nutritious. The dressing also helps to improve digestion. Choose the recipes that work best for you.

9. Mayonnaise with Apple Juice

Ingredients: 1 Tbs. walnuts, 1 Tbs. cold pressed olive oil, 3 Tbs. apple juice from "acid" apples.

Grind walnuts and mix them with the cold pressed olive oil and apple juice. May use blender on low speed.

10. Olive, Lemon, Onion Dressing

Ingredients: 2 Tbs. cold pressed olive oil, 1 Tbs. lemon juice, 1 Tbs. grated onion, 1 tsp. honey.

Mix all ingredients together and pour over the salad.

11. Sour Cream Tomato Dressing

Ingredients: 1 medium tomato, 2-3 Tbs. sour cream, 1 Tbs. lemon juice, 1 tsp. grated onion, 1 tsp. honey.

Peel the tomato and cut it into small pieces. Blend all ingredients in a blender on low speed.

12. Garlic Walnut Dressing

Ingredients: 4 Tbs. soaked walnuts, 2 cloves garlic, 1 Tbs. lemon juice.

Blend all ingredients in a blender on low speed for 5-10 seconds.

This dressing helps to release gas.

13. Honeyed Egg Yolk Dressing

Ingredients: 1 egg yolk, 1 Tbs. cold pressed olive oil, 1 Tbs. honey.

Mix well all ingredients and pour over salad. This dressing tastes best with salads which contain cabbage and carrots.

14. Veggie Sushi

Place a piece of nori on a sushi mat and layer the ingredients on top of the nori to about 1½ inches from the edge. Then roll the mat over tightly. Once rolled, seal the edges with a little lemon juice or water.

Ingredients for filling: 1) Avocado, mashed soaked pine nuts, mashed or sliced tomato, sliced or grated carrot, with the squeeze of a lemon. 2) Avocado, mashed or long-slivered cucumber, minced dill, with the squeeze of a lemon.

15. Vegetable Soup

Ingredients: 4 carrots, 1 tomato, 1 celery stick, 1 avocado, 1 garlic clove, 1 Tbs. Nama Shoyu, 1 green pepper, ½ onion, 1 cucumber, 3 Tbs. pine nuts.

Juice the carrots, tomato, and celery. Pour the juice in the blender. Add the avocado, garlic, and Nama Shoyu. Blend everything at medium speed until a uniform mass is formed.

Finely dice the pepper, onion, and cucumber. Put the diced vegetables into a soup tureen and add the pine nuts. Pour in the prepared liquid and stir.

16. Fruit Soup

Ingredients: 1/3 pineapple, 1-2 in. ginger, seedless grapes, 2 kiwis, 1 apple.

Wash and prepare the fruits. Make juice from the pineapple and ginger. Peel the kiwis and apple, and dice them into cubes of one cubic cm. Separate the grapes from the branch. Put the grapes, kiwi, and apples into a dish and pour in the juice. You can eat the soup immediately or let it soak for 20 minutes.

17. Meat, Chicken, and Fish

For individuals who eat meats and other animal products, it is best to eat these for lunch. Meat products require stronger digestive fires. At lunch time, the sun sends the most energy to Earth. This energy increases the acid in digestive juices needed to properly digest animal proteins. When you do eat meat or fish, it is best to start with raw vegetable salad.

Raw Vegetable Salad to Go with Meat: Cucumber, tomato, celery, spinach, lettuce, green onion.

Chicken or Fish.
Some Recipe Ideas:
Ingredients: Fish fillet or chicken (skinless, bone or boneless), 1 organic beet, 2 organic carrots, 1 onion, spices or seasoning to your taste (sea salt, pepper, dill, basil, paprika...).
Slice beets and carrots. Cut onions into thin half-circles. Place half of the beets, carrots, and onions on the bottom of a deep frying pan or backing dish. Put some spices over them. On top of the vegetable "bed" put chicken or fish. Put some seasoning over it. Put the rest of your beets, carrots, and onions on top, with a little more seasoning.
Cooking Instructions:
Two choices– stove top or oven.
If you choose to cook on the stove top in the frying pan, add about 3 oz. of water. Pour water on the sides not in the middle of your "pie." Cover the pan and set stove on High. As soon as the "pie" starts boiling (just a couple of minutes), set the stove on low and cook for about 30 minutes (for chicken, you might want to cook for 30-40 minutes).

If you decide to bake your dish, you don't have to add water, because meat and vegetables will produce their own juices. Cover your baking dish and set the oven 350. Cook for 35-50 minutes (longer for chicken). This meal will be very juicy and nutritious. It also has enough fiber to help the meat slide through your digestive system without causing any problems.

Please remember that meat or fish grown inorganically have artificial hormones, antibiotics and other harmful elements. These additives harm the endocrine system, kill the friendly bacteria and damage digestion. So please eat only organically grown fish, chicken, turkey, etc.

Meat and fish dishes are best absorbed with leafy greens and other low-carbohydrate vegetables, such as, cucumber, celery, tomato, green peppers (some consider these vegetables fruits).

Never eat animal proteins with carbohydrates, such as rice, breads, potatoes, etc. This wrong combination takes away from your body a lot of energy for digestion and creates an enormous level of toxic elements and gasses.

Another very important rule. When you eat meats, the proportion of vegetables to meat should be 4:1. In other words, eat **4 times more vegetables than meat.** Keep in mind that the total volume should not increase your **individual norm.** To learn how to calculate your individual norm for each meal, go to **page. 14.**

Other important factors to consider: After the meal, your **abdomen should not stick out,** but stay the same as it was before you ate. Also, your stomach should **not feel overloaded** and there should not be any pressure. On the contrary, you should feel light and that you could eat a little bit more. **You should also not feel tired or sleepy after a meal.** You should feel energy and willingness to be active.

The Third Chinese Wisdom

Give your supper to your enemies. As a rule, supper is the time when you can eat surrounded by your family gaining pleasure from the food and the socialization. Because of this, the preparation for supper frequently includes many dishes and much food. People fail to remember that it is **the supper that determines how well you will sleep, and how healthy and energized you will feel the next day.**

Due to daily human biorhythms, the digestive organs have very little energy in the evening. Overloading them with food means switching their function from digestion to the production of toxins. Food eaten at this time is digested slowly and poorly. **When we lie down to sleep, digestion nearly stops.**

On the other hand, the processes of fermentation, intoxication and parasite reproduction are activated in this situation. The stuffed stomach and small intestine block the functioning of the liver, the night organ. Bile collects in the liver and the gallbladder, and part of it is pressed into stones. Stagnant bile becomes aggressive, and after it gets to the small intestine, it irritates the walls, forms gas and fails in its job of digesting fats. When undigested fats absorb into blood, they stick to the walls of the vessels and clot there, creating the foundation of heart disease.

If you wish to be healthy, the supper must be small and easy to digest. **It is best if supper consists of drinking one or two cups of fresh vegetable juice.** For people with poor digestion, for the elderly, and for people who are ill, that is enough.

For those who are still young, healthy, and have good digestion, and for those who don't want to break the tradition of sitting down together for supper with the family (which *can be* extremely positive), this is the best time to eat warm, cooked or steamed food.

Heat plays a large role in good digestion. Raw, cold food would at this time be poorly digested and form a lot of gas (another reason to give your supper to your foe). At the same time, **small amounts** of warm food help digestion. Remember also the other things that help digestion: hunger, live enzymes, breathing through the right nostril, a walk while massaging your stomach after the meal, etc.

There is one more **important requirement for this food. It must be freshly prepared, using sparing preparation methods.** If you reheat yesterday's food, you lose a lot of valuable nutrition.

For food to be properly digested, you need living enzymes. Unfortunately, these are destroyed by cooking. A glass of fresh, live vegetable juice before the meal will supply the body with necessary enzymes. For people with poor digestion, this isn't enough; in addition they need to use digestive enzymes.

Thus, you may eat cooked food at supper, but skip supper altogether at least once a week. Monitor how you feel the next day.

Harmful Preparation Methods

Harmful preparation methods include: using high temperature over a long period of time; roasting, especially to charring; multiple reheatings of yesterday's or older food; using **microwave ovens**; and using high pressure, as in a pressure cooker. These techniques not only destroy useful nutrition, but also change them into poisons.

What Are Sparing Preparation Methods?

Sparing food preparation methods are ones that:
- Destroy only a limited amount of vitamins and minerals, and
- Don't change proteins, fats and carbohydrates into substances harmful to our bodies.

Here are the main methods known today:
- **Pre-soaking grain and beans to reduce cooking time.** Soak for 3-4 to 48 hours, depending on the kind of grain. If the soaking is prolonged, change the water every 8-10 hours.
- **Steaming the vegetables over a low flame.**
- **Using minimum temperature and minimum possible time.** The vegetables must still be chunky after preparation.
- **Cooking grains with cooling periods and repetitions of the cycle.** Example: For cooking a grain that requires a medium cooking time, bring it to a boil, lower the heat and cook for five minutes. Then turn off the heat and keep the grain under a lid for 15-30 minutes. Boil again, cook at low heat for 3-5 minutes. Then keep under a lid without a flame for 10-15 minutes, and the grain is done.
- **Wrapping.** This method is similar to the last one, but after turning off the heat, take the pot with beans or grain off the stove and wrap it with a blanket, a towel, or anything to preserve the heat. Usually, you need to keep the food wrapped for 30-60 or more minutes.
- **Keeping the food in a thermos.** Pour diced vegetables (carrot, onion, broccoli, zucchini), soft grains (buckwheat, or wheat), and slightly salty hot water into a thermos with a wide mouth. Keep in the thermos for 3-4 hours or more. When ready to eat, pour the contents of the thermos into a dish, add ghee and previously prepared thinly diced greens such as dill, cilantro, or garlic.

These methods are good for preparing supper dishes (like buckwheat or quinoa) or side dishes for lunch. Wash and dice vegetables and grain in the evening, put in a thermos, and pour in boiling water in the morning. The dish is ready three hours later.

Individuals who choose to eat a heavier breakfast, should have a very light supper. Your digestive organs worked very hard all day, so to give them some rest you may use recipes from the first part of breakfast (juices, smoothies, fruit salad). Those who chose to eat a mild, nutritious breakfast, may use the following recipes for supper. Still, keep in mind that supper should be very light, using only easy-to-digest foods in small amounts. If you came home late and **you don't have 3-4 hours before bedtime,** the best solution would be a glass of juice, herbal tea or plain kefir.

Supper Recipes

1. Raw Energy Soup

Ingredients:
1 zucchini
1 head broccoli
celery
½ onion
½ cup sunflower sprouts
1/4 cup pine nuts
½ cucumber

• Steam broccoli and zucchini for two to four minutes.

- In a separate pan, boil one quart plain, filtered water, adding a little sea salt or bouillon cubes from the health food store.
- Put the steamed broccoli and zucchini, together with the water which you used to steam them, into the blender.
- Add the hot, salty water and blend vegetables until you get a creamy consistency. This will be the base of the soup.
- Pour this solution in a separate pan.
- Add finely chopped celery, onion, cucumber, greens, and pine nuts.
- This soup combines the live, vital food products with a familiar, traditional taste.

2. World's Best Bread

Traditional yeast bread is bad for your health. It is especially bad for people who have a tumor, since the fermentation process in yeast activates the growth of the tumor. The recipe for this bread does not contain yeast. This bread contains enzymes, vitamins, and minerals in vital state. It also contains vital protein, fat, carbohydrates, B vitamins, and vitamin E, which is known as the vitamin of life. This bread tastes excellent, even to the infamous "picky eater." It can be made quickly and easily.

- Rinse thoroughly and dry 1-2 cups of organic whole wheat (spring soft wheat) or wheat alternative.
- Place wheat in a pan or other dish and add clean, filtered water to cover the wheat by one inch.
- Soak the wheat for 6-8 hours.
- Then pour out the water and cover with a towel to prevent the remaining moisture from evaporating and create a good sprouting conditions.

- In 12-24 hours small, white sprouts will appear. Put these wheat sprouts through a meat grinder.
- Add ½ onion, 2-3 cloves garlic, a piece of celery root, and put through the meat grinder again.
- Add sea salt to taste.
- Mix everything together and shape into small patties.
- Melt some butter in a frying pan. (If possible, use ghee instead of butter. Unlike cold pressed vegetable oil, ghee does not produce carcinogens.)
- Place patties in a frying pan, on moderate heat, for 1-2 minutes on each side.
- Then turn off the heat, cover and let stand for five minutes.
- Eat this bread while warm with vegetable salad, soup, or as a separate meal.

Variation: Sometimes you can add 1-2 eggs to the bread ingredients.

3. Grain "Cake"

- Choose three to four whole grains such as brown rice, millet, buckwheat, etc.
- Wash and dry each type of grain separately.
- On the bottom of a tall pan, place a layer of cabbage leaves.
- Place a thicker layer of rice (½ cup) on top of the cabbage leaves.
- Cover the rice with shredded carrots.
- Place a layer of millet (½ cup) over the carrots.
- Cover the millet with a layer of chopped onions.
- Place a layer of buckwheat over the onions.
- Cover the buckwheat with a layer of shredded zucchini. (Always finish this cake with a layer of vegetables.)

- Pour slightly salted, pure, cold water into the pan. The water should just cover the top layer of vegetables.
- Place the pan on the stove and bring to a boil.
- Reduce heat, cover, and continue simmering for 5-7 minutes.
- Turn off the heat and let sit for 20 minutes.
- Remove the cover and replace it with an upside down plate.
- Holding the plate securely, carefully turn over the pan onto the plate. Be careful not to burn yourself. This may require the help of another person.
- Slowly lift the pan. Underneath you will see a colorful "cake."

Variation: On one of the lower layers you can place sliced fish. The fish will absorb juice from this cake, and should have a wonderful taste. In this case you should cook the "cake" for twenty minutes, and let it stand for thirty more. Eat the fish first because fish is a protein and requires stronger gastric juices for digestion, which are on the bottom of the stomach. Then you can eat the grains.

4. Fruit Salad from Juice Pulp

- Make juice in a juicer from four carrots, two apples, and half a beet.
- Drink the juice and set aside the pulp for a fruit salad.
- To this pulp, add dried but soaked fruits such as raisins, apricots, plums, etc. (All fruits must be soaked the night before.)
- Add chopped walnuts, sour cream, or yogurt. You can also add fresh, shredded apples.

The food combination in this salad is not perfect, but it is a good cleanser for the colon.

5. Red Cleanser

- Cook or steam 1-2 red beets until soft. Cool the beets in cold water. (This will make them easier to peel.)
- Peel the beets and then shred them on a big grater.
- Add finely chopped green onion.
- Sprinkle with chopped walnuts, add 2-3 chopped garlic cloves, and pour on lemon juice.
- Add sea salt for taste and 1-2 tablespoons of cold pressed olive oil.

Note: All dishes which contain beets will color your bowel movements red. This is normal.

Note: Fresh juice from red beets will improve your blood consistency because it increases the number of red blood cells.

6. Soup from Sprouted Wheat

- Sprout wheat as you did for making bread.
- Cook vegetable soup from a variety of vegetables. You can use the principle of raw energy soup.
- When the soup is ready, add 4-5 tablespoons of sprouted wheat and let it stand for 10-15 minutes.
- Add finely chopped dill or parsley and mix.
- Then serve.

7. Balanced Grain Dish (Kasha)

For preparation of this dish, different kinds of **whole, uncut, unprocessed grains can be used**. This means that the grain will retain its own natural form, and also its own energetic values.

When grains or cereals are cut or ground into flour, they lose a great deal of energy. This is because energetic connections between molecules are broken and the energy of the grains dissipates. This happens despite the condition that processed grains do retain some nutritive material and quality. **The benefits from uncut, unground grains are much greater than the benefits from cut, processed grains.** For this dish, the following whole grains can be used: brown rice, whole wheat, buckwheat, quinoa, oats, etc.

Note of Caution: If grains are not stored correctly, molds can develop on them. If such grains are eaten, the bacterial balance in the colon could be damaged and, for example, candida may develop. Also note that improperly stored wheat can develop an ergot which has a crude but effective version of lysergic acid diethylmide (LSD). This will ruin your day, maybe your life.

To avoid this problem, put grains in a dry, hot frying pan for 2-3 minutes. Stir constantly to make sure that the grains do not lose their primary color. Keeping grains on the hot, dry frying pan for this amount of time not only destroys the molds, but also helps to improve absorption and assimilation of the grain starches in the human digestive system.

- Remove the grains from the pan. Put them in a cold, dry container or dish to cool a little.
- Then, it is important to wash the grains thoroughly.
- Soak the grains in clean cold water (1 cup grains for 2-3 cups of water). Soak rice for 8 hours, oats for 12 hours, and wheat and buckwheat for 4 hours. Soaking the grains activates their own processes of sprouting. Even though sprouting does not actually happen, the activation of enzymes, vitamins and minerals increases, and cooking time decreases significantly. This promotes better preservation of nourishing elements.
- It is good to add cut or shredded steamed vegetables, such as carrots, celery, onion, or broccoli to the already cooked

grains. Also, it is a good, healthy idea to add freshly cut garlic, cold pressed olive oil or ghee, some green leaves of parsley or dill, and a little sea salt.

8. Red Vegetable Soup (Classic Russian Borshch)

Ingredients:
3 organic potatoes with the skin
1 organic carrot
1 zucchini
½ red pepper
1 red beet
½ white cabbage
1 qt. water to boil
1 glass tomato juice
½ lemon, juiced
Sea salt
Parsley leaves
Dill leaves
2-3 med cloves garlic
1 tsp. per serving of sour cream

- Prepare the potatoes, carrot, zucchini, pepper, and beet by cleaning, drying, and shredding each on a large grater.
- Chop the cabbage very finely or shred it with a special blade.
- Drop the prepared vegetables into boiling water. (This action automatically decreases the temperature of the water.)
- Wait until the water boils again, turn off the heat, cover, and let stand for 20-30 minutes or more.
- Then add tomato and lemon juice, and a little sea salt as desired.

- Add finely chopped fresh leaves from parsley and dill, and fresh cloves of garlic.
- Stir all together one more time, and then serve hot.
- Drop one teaspoon sour cream into each bowl.

Monodiet

Very often people disturb their digestion so badly that they don't have the ability to digest even simple dishes. To solve this problem and restore digestive function, it is necessary to cleanse the digestive system and give the digestive organs some rest. The most efficient yet simple way to gain such rest is through the monodiet.

The monodiet is a way of eating in which, during one whole meal, you eat only one kind of product, and you change the choice of product from meal to meal over a period of three days to two weeks and more.

The monodiet was the normal diet for primitive people because when a person climbed a tree to eat a meal, there was no mixed fruit dish at the top of the tree. They could eat only one kind of fruit without any mixing.

During the monodiet, the system spends minimum energy for digestion. If you feel you need the monodiet to improve your digestion, you can start with something like this example:

Day One Breakfast: Apples
    Lunch: Plums
    Dinner: Carrots
Day Two Breakfast: Strawberries
    Lunch: Cabbage
    Dinner: Brown rice cooked with water
Further Days in Similar Fashion

If you feel hungry between meals, drink more water. Besides calming your hunger, this will help to cleanse your system. If your digestion has been poor, the fact that you feel hunger is very positive because hunger will activate the stomach and stomach buds to release more and stronger digestive juices. So don't be afraid to feel hunger.

When you on the monodiet, you can eat more than three times a day because the time required to assimilate the food is shorter during this way of eating.

The next way to improve and wake up your digestion is through fasting. Those who regularly do cleansing of the digestive organs and fasting, even short fasting for 1-3 days, do not suffer from poor digestion.

For instructions on performing a short fast, see Book 3 of this series, *Healing through Cleansing*. For how to accomplish and correctly exit from long fasting, see my book, *Eight Steps to Perfect Health*.

Approximate Food Schedule

- **Breakfast:** Herbal Tea, Fruit (in season) or Fruit Juice
- **Lunch:** Vegetable juice. Raw vegetable salad (spinach, tomato, cucumber, onions, etc. *see page 45 for examples*) plus: baked potato <u>or</u> fish, or organic chicken. You should have 70% of the salad and only 30% of the other.
- **Dinner:** Vegetable juice or Herbal tea. Raw vegetable salad or a vegetable soup. Whole grain porridge (brown rice, millet, buckwheat, etc) cooked on water (not milk) with slightly steamed or grilled vegetables (carrots, onions, broccoli, cauliflower, etc) *see page 59 for details.*

Note: Some individuals, depending on their work schedules or other individual characteristics, could switch breakfast and dinner *(eat grain with vegetables in the morning and fruit in the evening)*.

Conclusion

The diet plays an essential role in preserving and restoring health. Because of this, we want to eat the best quality food available.

People often think that food is simply a source of energy to keep them going and alive. **Food is more than that. Food is a source of energy and matter for our cells, organs, and systems.** Our bodies do not build these out of pure energy, or "out of thin air." If we want our cells, organs and systems to be as healthy as possible then the material we use to build them must be the highest quality available. Food must be organic, prepared correctly, and eaten according to proper dietary principles. When there are disorders in the body such as illness, etc., no matter what the cause (stress, overwork, low grade poisoning, auto-intoxication, etc.) you should temporarily stop eating.

Do a colon cleansing and then fast. (See Book 1.) The removal of accumulated waste in the colon helps free the immune system to concentrate more resources on the disorder. Fasting frees up additional energy for the immune system by the body not having to spend precious energy on digestion. "Hot" water (do not burn yourself!) with lemon juice, calming teas from mint, dandelion or camomile, and a little fresh, non-sweet, filtered juice is all the body needs. Then it will quickly heal itself.

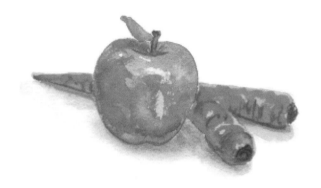

Diet for Various Purposes

Different situations call for different solutions. For instance, the person who is very ill might need to react to the food Americans usually serve on celebration days in a different way than the person would who has no major health problems and eats a healthy diet almost every day.

Diet for Healing from Disease

If someone has a health problem, a strict diet is recommended, especially if the illness is serious. In this case, it

65

is better to follow a 100% raw diet, and the best raw diet for healing is juice therapy, that is, using only raw fresh juices. The duration of such a diet, otherwise called Juice Fasting, can be 3-30 days or more, depending on the problem to be solved. After completing this fast, you should strictly follow the rules for how to break the fast, which are described in my book, *Eight Steps to Perfect Health*. If the problem is not solved completely with this fast, then in a month's time intensive juice therapy may be repeated. Such fasting could be repeated 2-4 times, depending on the problem. If juice therapy lasts more than three days, it requires professional control and regular Colon Cleanses according to detailed instructions in my book, *Eight Steps to Perfect Health*.

Related to this healing diet is the mono-diet. This means eating only one type of product, for example watermelons, for 3-7 days and more. If the problem is not too serious, one can eat different types of raw foods in limited amounts, considering proper food combining, and choosing not more that 3-4 ingredients at one time. You should be sure to choose food products which do not give you a lot of gas; otherwise you may undermine your digestion and get more toxins than nutrients.

Usually if you have a health problem, your own experience may not be enough. In this case it is better to seek professional consultation. You should remember that in many serious cases, eating only raw, living food is not enough. It is better to combine a healing diet with deep internal body cleansing and exercises such as Yoga and conscious relaxation of muscles and internal organs to release blockages and stress tensions and to open energy channels. It is also important to include special breathing to balance the energy field or aura. I will describe this type of breathing in my next book, which will be about breathing.

A healing diet could be used not only for healing from disease but also for prevention. When you practice prevention without waiting until you feel ill, this is the best way to preserve your health. A prevention diet can be done about four times a year for 3-6 weeks, or constantly during the whole life if old habits and societal traditions don't hinder you.

If you have been healed from disease or are just plain healthy, it is not necessary to follow a 100% raw diet for 365 days in a year. If you try to force yourself through a long period of resisting what you want, you will do a long violation on your body, more dangerous to you than eating a little cooked food.

Diet for Every Day

People who advocate a raw diet claim that, after cooking, the product becomes completely unuseable for the system. If this were true, our civilization would have been extinct long ago. Not everything is killed in cooking. In cooked food there still could be something of which we have no knowledge. Today's knowledge is not enough to give a good answer to this question.

If we applied to statistics among centenarians, people who lived in the previous centuries, we can meet people who lived 120 or 170 years. When I researched about their diet, I found among them almost nobody who was completely on a raw diet, only one man I know of who was on a raw diet since the age of 50 and lived to be 119 years old. That was Norman Walker, but in addition to this diet, he regularly did Colon Cleansing during his whole life. I think this combination played important roles. He also drank a large amount of raw fresh juices.

When we age, digestion slows down, and digesting solid food becomes more difficult. Our body has a chronic deficiency in nutrients. Raw fresh juices, smoothies, and other types of liquid diet digest much easier and give our system essential nutrients without wasting energy for digestion. Centenarians from the mountains use in their diet a lot of **fresh,** wild greens which contain much life power and are filled with vitamins, minerals, etc. Other items which also played an important role in their health are the clean mountain air and the moderate physical activities. Whatever cooked food they ate was simple, and of course there were no dishes from McDonald's. I have given simple and healthy recipes for cooked food in this book and also in the book, *Unique Method of Colon Rejuvenation.*

Let's put all products in a row according to their value for health. What will be in first place? Of course, air or oxygen is product number one. Without oxygen we cannot live more than a few minutes. In the second place will be water, and solid food comes only in third place because without solid food we can survive 30-100 days and more.

Therefore, right breathing with clean air which feeds the blood cells with oxygen is much more important than whether you are 100% raw foodist or only 80%.

If you are sick, don't let anybody turn you from your way until you get healthy. Everybody may understand your need to be different right now. But if you are healthy, be moderate because food is not only food for the body; it is also food for the soul, and the soul doesn't need any vitamins or enzymes. The best foods for the soul are a good mood and positive emotions. If cooked food can give you this joy, you can allow yourself to eat it **sometimes.** Again, be moderated because prolonged wrong diet can damage the soul.

As I said before, raw foods contain enzymes which are important for digestion, and **raw foods should take precedence in our diet, not less than 60% of the total amount, and even more.** When you mix a diet of raw and cooked foods, you still need to follow the main principles of healthy eating. If your body and soul agree with a 100% raw food diet, then follow your intuition, and God bless you.

Diet for Celebration and Soul

The casual raw food diet should be simple and easy to digest, but a raw diet can be not only casual. There are many interesting recipes which can make raw food into celebration food. These recipes you can find in many books about the raw food diet.

In our days there are some restaurants where you can buy only raw dishes. There you can order dishes which look like regular dishes (pizza, lasagna, and others) but they are made from only raw vegetables, greens, and sprouts, nuts, and seeds.

There are also healthy restaurants where you can order raw and cooked food. For some people these restaurants will be more convenient because they go there not only to eat but to spend time around family and friends. It could happen that not everybody in your group can eat 100% raw food. If you go to a strict raw food restaurant, your friends probably won't have another choice, and if they don't like it they can feel uncomfortable. The idea is to provide choices, but everybody needs to choose for himself what to take. If you are around people who accept raw food, then it will be more interesting to spend time around these people in the restaurant of raw food. Do not overeat. You need to remember that fancy recipes of raw food could be difficult for some people to digest, the same as cooked celebration food.

If you eat something with good taste but difficult to digest, eat only a small amount of this food and on the next day give your body a rest and drink only juices or water. It will be even better if you do a Colon Cleansing on that day. This will allow your body to mobilize its energy, eliminate toxins, and be coming back to balance.

Conclusion: On a celebration you may allow yourself more freedom than on a daily basis, but a celebration diet does not mean 100% traditional heavy food, which may make you feel terrible on the next day. The major amount of your food, 70% or even 80%, should still be your regular healthy food, with only 30% or 20% being something special.

To learn more about unique cleansing procedures done in our center, please visit our website at
www.koyfmancenter.com

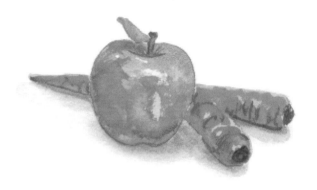

Desserts

Why We Like Desserts

In a regular diet, the eating of dessert is a very casual habit. The roots of this dessert habit lie in long centuries of tradition, taught by parents to their children from babyhood.

Another reason for the dessert eating habit very often comes from the unbalanced diet. With such a diet in the stomach, one often feels discomfort and the hope is that dessert will make it better.

If you improve your diet and follow all the principles of healthy eating, such as right food order during one meal, right food combining, timing, and other principles described in this book, you will get rid of the unhealthy habit of eating desserts.

You will be glad you did because desserts slow down and destroy digestion, poison the system, and increase your weight.

On the other hand, we cannot ignore the fact that, for many people, dessert is a pleasant part of the meal and people wait for it with eager expectation. After they eat the dessert they feel guilty. Feeling guilty is as dangerous for the system as the dessert itself because feeling this way is a negative emotion which brings to the system many other problems.

Dessert from raw food is less dangerous than traditional desserts, but is still not ideal food. Raw food desserts often contain a lot of sugar, fat, protein, and wrong combinations of ingredients, but are a little better than traditional desserts, especially if you eat them in small quantities and not too often.

I will give you some recipes and ideas, and you can create your own recipes by exchanging ingredients. Remember you need to follow good hygiene, which means careful cleaning of all products which you will use.

Raw Foods Hygiene and Healthy Flora

Some people claim that raw foods have on their surfaces friendly flora which help digestion. In ideal situations, this would be true. However, if you start thinking about what, besides friendly bacteria, is on the surface of the industrial product, you will consider what things these products go through in the processes of growth, harvest, transport, storage, and display, who handles them, and what animals might have been in the boxes. Then you will also realize that the dirt on the surface of the raw product may contain mold, parasite eggs, excrement from rats, excrement from other animals brought in as fertilizer, and chemicals that accumulate in the land from previous years. So you will realize how unhealthy the method is to eat the dirt in order to get friendly bacteria from the surface of the raw food product.

How much better it is to clean everything carefully and to get our friendly bacteria from acidophilus, cultured vegetables, kefir, etc. In a clean internal environment, our systems can create the friendly flora from fresh and clean products.

Eating uncleansed products can lead to infections, illnesses, and multiplying dangerous parasites. Even if you test for parasites, and don't find them, you cannot be sure they are not in your system. Parasites live in the human system so shyly that we cannot know for sure whether they are present or not for awhile. If you are not following the rules of hygiene and cleansing procedures, the number of parasites and their eggs will increase and there will come the time when they can be found. If you have a strong immune system, that time will be longer; if your immune system is weak, the time required to know the presence of parasites will be shorter. For more detail about how to fight parasites and prevent their invasion, read Book 3 of this series, *Healing through Cleansing*.

Raw Food Recipes for Desserts

1. Ice Cream

You can make ice cream on a base of fruit juices such as apple, orange, and pineapple. You can also experiment with others.

Ingredients:
1 orange
1 raw pineapple

1 mango
4-5 frozen strawberries
½ c. raw cashews

- In a Champion juicer, make 2-3 cups of juice from the orange and pineapple.
- Poor the juice into the Vita-Mix, and add the mango, strawberries, and cashews.
- Blend for 1 minute.
- Poor this cocktail into ice cube trays and put into freezer.
- When the cubes are frozen, use a Champion juicer, exchanging the metal screen for a plastic blind that comes with the juicer. Put the juice cubes in the entrance funnel and process as usual.

This ice cream comes out of the Champion juicer with a good taste and texture. If you like it chocolate color, you can add carob or dates together with the juice ice cubes.

You can make ice cream from only two ingredients by freezing mango pieces and strawberries to put through the Champion juicer in the same way.

One-ingredient ice cream can be made by cutting banana into small pieces before freezing and then juicing.

You can exchange plastic bags zipped shut in place of the ice cube trays. You will probably need to use the Vita-Mix for the final processing of the larger frozen mass.

You can exchange the mango for peaches, strawberries for other berries. You can create your own favorite recipes.

2. Raw Cake

To make a raw cake, you will need a food processor or electric meat grinder. The meat grinder could be used for

74

soaked nuts and soaked dried fruits. Using soaked nuts and soaked dried fruits is even healthier than using them dried. If you use a food processor, you will need "C" blades to make a flour-like dough from the dried nuts fruits.

Ingredients:
1 c. nuts: walnuts, cashews, almonds, etc.
1 c. dried fruits: raisins, dates, etc.
1 apple or other fruit, peeled and cut into small pieces
1 banana
Few drops lemon juice

- Clean the nuts and soak them overnight or at least 4 hours.
- Clean the dried fruits and soak them for 30-60 minutes.
- Process the nuts and dried fruits through an electric meat grinder, mixing to make a flour-like dough-ball.
- Use part of the mixture to form and shape a "crust" about 1/4" thick and place on bottom of cake dish or pan.
- Peel and core an apple or other raw fruit and cut it into small pieces.
- Cover crust with a 1/4" layer of apple pieces.
- Make another "crust" and lay it on top of apples.
- Cover second crust with banana cut into small pieces.
- On the bananas sprinkle a few drops of lemon juice for variety in taste.
- Put another layer of "crust" on top of the bananas.
- Now we will make a cream for this cake

Cream:
1-2 handfuls of pine nuts
Water to cover pine nuts
1-2 Tbs. natural honey

- Put pine nuts in Vita-Mix.
- Add water to reach the same level as the nuts.
- Add honey.
- Blend to the consistency of thick cream.
- Pour cream over the cake and garnish with fresh berries, strawberries, pieces of walnuts, etc.
- If you want a chocolate color, you can add carob or dates to the cream.

3. Raw Candy

Ingredients:
Wheat (soft wheat spring berries) or wheat alternative
Dried fruits, like figs, raisins, etc.

- Sprout the wheat as in the recipe for the World's Best Bread.
- Soak the dried fruits for one hour.
- Process the wheat and dried fruits through a meat grinder or food processor using "C" blades.
- From the resulting mass, shape candy in the forms of balls, cones, cubes, etc. To help shape cones you can use special small drinking cups.
- You may want to place the candy pieces in a re-usable candy box to store in refrigerator or give as a gift.

Variations:
- You can hollow out spaces on the insides of these shapes to hide interesting things.
- In the balls, you can put grapes, nuts, or berries.
- In the cones, you can use a special syringe to inject ice cream or liquid cocktail.

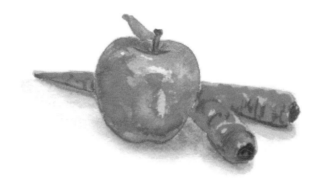

Weight Loss and Healing Program

There are many programs for weight loss through dieting. Modern Americans are inundated with advertisements on television, radio, magazines, newspapers, etc., trumpeting the "great success" a particular weight loss program provides. There is one thing these weight loss programs all have in common: money. The proprietors want you to buy their program so they can make a profit.

Some of the basic types of these unhappy, sales-driven weight loss programs are as follows.

- Many programs exclude fats from the diet; they are based on the consumption of fat-free products.

- Others require a diet consisting almost exclusively of protein, fish, meat, eggs three times a day, with very little vegetable food.
- A third kind of program limits nothing in the diet, not fats, nor flour, nor sweets. In this case, you must regularly consume special tablets that neutralize the consumed calories.
- The fourth kind of program provides a diet consisting not of food but of various dried and powdered natural food products to be mixed with water. This soup is supposed to neutralize your hunger.

The first program makes no account for the quality or freshness of food, the presence in it of artificial chemicals, or care for correct combinations, etc. Further, the technology of fat removal alters the products so much that they become more harmful to your health than the fat itself.

The second program is not for those who have low acidity in gastric juice. Although many people lose weight and feel fine on this program, it is unhealthy and boring to eat a diet of animal protein for a long time.

The third program also doesn't lead to health. On one hand, it lets you eat all kinds of garbage that can't be used to build healthy cells and organs. On the other hand, the use of tablets to neutralize calories disturbs, both immediately and permanently, the chemistry of digestion—and that's a sure way to disease.

The fourth program is profit-driven. It is laughable to think that pills, and dried and powdered products can replace (for a significant period of time) food made by nature. Only those who can taste the profits from the sale of these products can sing of their product's great taste, healthiness, and effectiveness. People who only consume the products would soon get tired of them and abandon the products. That is why distributing companies try to interest everyone in not only consuming their products but also in making money by bringing in an increasing number of new people to consume the products and on whom their income depends. This is a perfect system for brainwashing innocent people with false information on nutrition and a strong desire to put profit first.

After a person loses the desired amount of weight with such diets, he or she typically returns to his or her former "diet." Wait a minute. Wasn't this the "diet" that caused the weight gain in the first place? Don't people realize what is about to happen? As they return to their customary manner of eating they begin to regain the excess weight that they have just lost. The typical problem is that this time they regain even more excess weight than they had in the first place.

On these poorly designed weight loss programs, people lose not only weight, but also good health. This is because as the returning excess weight appears, so does the increased chance for disease.

The central idea of a weight loss program should not be merely the loss of excess fat for a good figure. **Instead, all weight loss programs *should* put their primary emphasis on maximizing health by losing dangerous weight that increases the chance of disease.** What good was that fad diet once they close the coffin lid?

The greatest foundation for any diet should be that your diet is one you can eat for the rest of your life for the purpose of maximum health, i.e., longevity and quality of life. Such a diet is *not* a temporary plan for short term goals. Instead it is a long term **strategy** that obtains and maintains optimum health through a **lifestyle diet**. Only this kind of diet, which accounts for all the principles of good nutrition, can keep your weight under control and give you the best possible health. By following the rules of nutrition described in this series of books, you will do more than normalize your weight. You will maximize your quality and length of your life.

Please realize and remember that a significant part of most people's excess weight is toxins stored in the body. In some people, the deposits in the large intestine alone weigh 10-70 pounds. So cleansing the colon and other organs will help you lose quite a bit of harmful, toxic weight. Then, correct and healthy nutrition will build healthy cells where toxic cells once struggled for life.

For those who want to accelerate their weight loss, I wish to offer a program that includes both weight loss and increased protection from disease.

You may want to return to this program several times per year to get rid of the toxins that enter the body constantly, weaken it and create the conditions for the development of disease.

This program will also correct the bad habits your taste buds have gotten into. (They have been hanging out with bad foods, you know.) Once you get rid of the bad habits that contribute to the desire to eat bad foods you will develop the desire to eat only healthy foods. When the craving for unhealthy food returns, it means that it is time to repeat this program for several days.

To complete this program of loss of weight, enhanced disease protection, and freedom from bad eating habits, you will need a blender and a juicer, plus organic fruits, vegetables, and berries.

An important condition of this program is that it should be completed in conjunction with colon cleansing. Colon cleansing will give you energy and the feeling of lightness, and will speed up weight loss due to the removal of the toxic weight on the walls of the colon.

Program 1

Over the course of a month, you will eat according to the principles described in this book. Every third day, you only drink fresh juices during the day, and in the evening you may eat Fruit Cocktail or raw Vegetable Soup. (Recipes included in the previous chapter.) In one month this will give you ten unloading days. Simple, direct and effective.

Program 2

Over the course of 10 days, you will eat according to the program that I use while breaking a fast and switching to a raw diet. Then you will take a 10-day break and eat healthy food according to this book's recipes. Then you spend another 10 days on the fast-breaking diet.

Day One

Breakfast   **Fruit Smoothie**
1. In Champion Juicer, make juice from oranges, grapefruit, apples, pineapples, or any two of these in combination.
2. Put pulp through the juicer 2-4 times to make juice thicker and more nutritional.
3. Pour juice into Vita-Mix and add pieces of mango or papaya.
4. Add 3-4 ice cubes made from pure water.
5. Blend 15-30 seconds.
6. If this is too sweet, squeeze some lemon juice into it.

7. Drink.
After breakfast, continue as on fast. Drink juices, herbal tea, and water.

Day Two

Breakfast Same as Day One.

Lunch **Vegetable Soup**
1. In Champion Juicer, make juice from carrots and celery.
2. Put pulp through the juicer 1-2 times to make juice thicker and more nutritional.
3. Pour juice into Vita-Mix and add pieces of tomato, cucumber, green pepper, or zucchini, or a combination of 2-3 of these. Juice should always cover the pieces.
4. Blend and drink.
Continue to drink juices, herbal tea, and water as on the fast.

Day Three

Breakfast **Fruit Smoothie**
Same as Day One, but add to the Fruit Smoothie half a bunch of spinach in the blender.

Lunch **Vegetable Soup**
Same as Day Two, but add to the Vegetable Soup some kale leaves in the blender.

Dinner **Vegetable Juice**

In any vegetable juice add 1 tsp. cold pressed flax seed oil. Between meals, drink water, herbal tea, and some juice.

Day Four

Breakfast **Fruit Smoothie**
Same as Day Three, but add to the Fruit Smoothie 1-2 Tbs. frozen fruits and 1 tsp. cold pressed flax seed oil in the blender.

Lunch **Vegetable Soup**
Same as Day Three, but add to the Vegetable Soup 1/3 ripe avocado and 1 medium-sized clove of garlic in the blender.

Dinner **Nut Milk**
1. Use 1-2 Tbs. soaked nuts: cashew, walnut, or others. If almond, it is recommended to peel the skin.
2. Put nuts into Vita-mix.
3. Add 1 cup apple juice and ½ cup pure water plus 3-4 pitted dates and 3-4 ice cubes.
4. Blend 60 seconds.
5. Strain.
6. Chew your juices for 20 seconds.

Day Five Same as Day Four, but add 2 tsp. cold pressed flax seed oil for breakfast and ½ ripe avocado for lunch.

Day Six

Breakfast
Fruit Salad
Cut apples, kiwi, grapes, and put on a plate. Pour over them the Fruit Smoothie made from the recipe on Day Five.

Lunch
Vegetable Soup
Cut tomatoes, a cucumber, some green onion and bell pepper, and pour over the Vegetable Soup made from the recipe on Day Five.

Dinner
Nut Milk
Use 2-3 Tbs. nuts that have been soaked 8-12 hours. Blend, strain, and chew the same as on Day Four.

Day Seven through Day Ten

Continue the same as on Day Six.

Then you can carefully add other foods and pay attention to the reaction of your digestion.

Program 3

Over the course of 14-21 days, you will drink only fresh fruit and vegetable juices that you make yourself with your juicer, pure water, and herbal teas all day long. (See recipes in the previous chapter.) Then, in the evening, between 5 and 7 p.m., you eat one small meal (vegetable salad, or vegetable soup, or cooked grain with stewed vegetables, or fruit, berries, watermelon, or melon). Then, if hunger returns, drink herbal tea. (For sweetening, use a little honey or, even better, stevia, although it is best to use no sweeteners.) If, after the program, you aren't satisfied with your results in terms of weight loss, you can repeat everything 10-15 days later. This program may be called a partial fast. Do not forget to do 1-2 sessions a week of Colon Cleansings during this fast.

Program 4

This is the most serious program, not only for weight loss but also for powerful treatment of diseases. This program is conducted under the guidance of a specialist, with the majority of it actually done by you yourself. For those who have serious health problems, this program is best. It is always helpful to combine your own effort with the expertise of a professional.

The essence of this program is that you completely switch to water, fresh fruit and vegetable juices, herbal teas, and, if you wish, vegetable decoctions. You can stay on this diet for 2-4 weeks, sometimes more. Practically, this is what is called **juice fasting.**

Weight Loss, Healing and Rejuvenation Program

Preparation for the Fast

To make fasting successful and yield the best results, it is necessary to do all the steps properly.

Three days prior to beginning the fast, stay on a strict cleansing vegetarian diet: fruits, soaked dried fruits, fresh fruit and vegetable juices, fresh salads, soups, grains, small amounts of nuts and seeds soaked in water for 4-8 hours.

Entering the Fast

Often those who don't understand deeply the processes that happen in the body during fasting begin fasting without any special care on entry. This is not wise. During fasting, the system does not stop feeding; it simply reorients during the fast to internal feeding. If the fasting begins without complete cleansing of the digestive system, then the body will spend a long time feeding and poisoning itself on the leftovers and toxins which remain there. Such fasting is difficult for the person fasting. You may feel weakness, dizziness, nausea, or heart palpitations.

When fasting begins with a full cleansing of the digestive system including the stomach, small intestine, and colon, then the body already on the second day turns to cell feeding. Old and ill cells go through the digestive process and are "digested." The healthy cells are left alone; the digestive process does not touch them.

In the fire of internal digestion burns away toxic mucus, excessive fat, tumors, etc. The fast flushes from the system everything that weakens and poisons it: medicine, chemicals, artificial colors, heavy metals, toxic bile, stones, parasites, etc.

During such fasting the body gets rid of the worst and most dangerous weight, the weight of toxins. Losing toxic weight (10-70 lbs.) improves the immune system. In the body begins the healing and rejuvenation processes

The liver plays a very important role during the fast in neutralizing toxins. So if the liver is cleaner, it is easier to go through the fast. **A day of Liver Cleansing could be an entrance to the fast.**

So, if we combine Liver Cleansing and cleansing of the whole digestive system, which we can reach through Small Intestine Cleansing, such fasting will be the more effective, and you can go through the fast with ease and comfort. It is not quite so perfect, but still possible, to start the fast with a mere Colon Cleansing.

Important Procedures During the Fast

During the fast, and through the first week when you break the fast, you may do any of the following combinations of the following procedures. **The more procedures you do the more toxins you release and the better you feel.**
• Colon Cleansing.
• Colon Cleansing with Internal Organ Massage.
• Colon Cleansing with sauna.
• Full body cleansing massage with a Colon Cleansing and sauna.

Doing the Fast Itself

This is a sample of a fasting schedule during the day. Depending on your schedule, your work and any personal health problem, you can change it. Just keep in mind the main principles. (See section below entitled, "Important Principles of Fasting.")

7:00 a.m.   a.   In the morning after waking up, drink 1 to 2 glasses of warm, distilled water plus 1 tsp. strained lemon juice. Add to the water a pinch of sea salt for neutralizing toxins which accumulate in the stomach during the night.

b. Warm or contrast shower without soap.

c. Dry skin brush massage, 3 to 5 minutes.

d. Light morning exercise, 10 to 15 minutes.

e. Outside walking, 20 minutes to 1 hour, with cleansing breathing technique (described in the book, *Healing through Cleansing, Book 1,* in the chapter on the lungs).

9:00 a.m. Big cup of warm herbal mint tea.

11:00 a.m. Fruit juice: ½ cup juice (citrus, such as grapefruit, lemon, or orange, or apple) in ½ cup distilled water. **All juices on a fast must be strained**. This will prevent the stomach from having to work during the fast by digesting small food particles. It will also help to rest the colon. The juice will be absorbed directly by the small intestines.

1:00 p.m. Vegetable juice (strained): 1 to 2 glasses.
*60% choice of 2-3 kinds of green juices: celery, romaine lettuce, spinach, kale, cucumber, mustard and other greens.
*40% juice from carrots, apples or pineapples.

3:00 p.m. Warm herbal tea from rose hips or fasting tea.

5:00 p.m. a. Apple/beet juice: 4 apples plus 1/4 beet.
b. 1 to 2 glasses clean, distilled water.

7:00 p.m.   1 to 2 cups warm, strained vegetable broth (recipe below).

9:00 p.m.   Warm herbal tea with camomile. May add ⅓ to ½ tsp. honey dissolved in tea. If you have yeast, do not use honey.

Walking before going to bed, 30 minutes. This is NOT power walking but strolling *for relaxation,* so do not walk too fast.

Warm shower without soap. This is to increase circulation not for exterior cleanliness. Shower or bathe for exterior cleanliness at a different time.

10:00-11:00 p.m.   Go to bed no later than this time.

Recipe for Vegetable Broth:

Base: 1. Two big organic potatoes cut into cubes (1 cm.).
       2. One glass shredded carrot.
       3. One glass shredded beet.
       4. One glass shredded celery sticks or root.

Can be added:
       1. One-half glass cut onion.
       2. Roots of parsley.
       3. Beet top.

Cover this with good clean water or previously distilled water, 1 or 2 cm. above the vegetables. Bring to a boil, then continue to simmer on low heat for 30 minutes. Turn off heat. Add upper green parts of beet, dill and parsley. Let stand for

30 minutes. Strain. While it is still warm, drink 1 or 2 eight-ounce cups. Put the rest in the refrigerator.

Notice: All teas, juices, broths must be strained and warm or cool (never cold) when drunk.

Important Principles of Fasting

1. Wear clean clothes because they will help to accumulate more toxins from the skin. So change your clothes every single day. The underwear is the most important article of clothing here.
2. Use underwear made of natural fibers, not synthetic materials. Synthetic clothes accumulate negative electricity which can destroy body energies.
3. Wear extra clothing to stay warm since you might feel cold during a fast. If you have more clothes and don't feel cold, you save more energy for healing rather than wasting it for heating.
4. Before drinking anything, rinse your mouth with water, or water plus baking soda, or water and lemon juice.
5. During the day, try to find the time for walking 1 to 2 hours. During fasting, our bodies need more oxygen to neutralize the toxins.
6. Do a dry brush massage every morning and possibly every evening for 5-10 minutes.
7. Get some light exercise.
8. Try to stay calm, concentrate on yourself, not reacting to anything around you.
9. Try to find time for resting with warm water bottle on the right side for 30 to 60 minutes to heat your liver. (It will help your liver to detoxify itself and your whole body).
10. At any time, when you feel thirst, hunger or discomfort, drink distilled water.

11. Take a warm bath at least every other day, better every day. During fasting, the body cools down without food to warm it up. A warm bath helps to warm it up, stimulate circulation for toxin removal and to soak the toxins out. If you are doing a warm bath, you may skip #10 above.

12. Call the Center any time you feel you need support or help.

13. Don't break the fast without consulting with the Center. Breaking the fast when you are not feeling well involves a special program.

Tips to Remember

• Fasting cleanses and rejuvenates the whole body down to the cellular level.

• During fasting some people feel a slight discomfort, plus "flashbacks" to the feelings of old diseases and disorders, weakness, etc., as their stored remnants work themselves out. But all of this is for a short period of time, tolerable, and so much easier than the diseases themselves. These are called "healing events."

• If you feel bad, drink a cup of water with a pinch of sea salt to neutralize toxins (people who don't have yeast can add 1/3 teaspoon of honey).

• The benefits fasting brings are so amazing that it is worth the challenge.

• Look at this struggle as your fight with the sickness living inside you. In this fight you must win.

Caution: After you complete your fast, it is very important to break the fast correctly. Incorrect exiting

from the fast may destroy all the benefits from your efforts as well as your health.

To find out how to break a fast, read the chapter entitled, "Detailed Instructions for Exiting the Fast" in my book, *Eight Steps to Perfect Health.*

"Within a Day Pain Was Gone"

I came to the Center because I had pain in my right pelvic region which radiated to my lower back. It started about two and a half months ago, and I did nothing because the pain was minor. It intensified over time, however, and I got scared. I began a series of colonic irrigations, but I did not clean up my diet. Although I do not eat meat or sugar, I did sometimes eat white flour and dairy. The pain continued. Finally, after over a month of coming here, I decided to eat as Dr. Koyfman told me I must eat-millet, steamed veggies, a little fruit, water, and nothing else. Within a day, pain which had plagued me was gone. I've had no pain for three days, my pelvic sonogram was normal, and urinalyses was normal. I will keep you posted. Later, after moving to Seattle, Washington Cathy writes:

Dear Dr. Koyfman,

I don't know how to begin this note because it is so hard for me to say goodbye. To say that you have made an impact on my life is such an understatement-you've changed my life. I will remember the lessons you've taught me and will use the techniques for the rest of my life, I'm sure. Hopefully my husband and daughter will too. Please know that there is a very grateful and healthier family in Seattle, thinking of you with respect and love.

- - - **Cathy M.** - - -
Seattle, WA

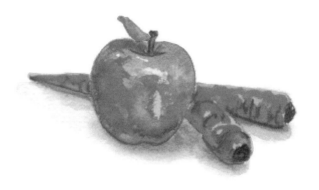

Support from Higher Forces

Disease Caused by a False World View

A large portion of human disease is caused by a false world view, by wrong choices regarding what is most important to us in this life and what is secondary.

Example 1

Often, we choose some famous or successful person whom we think we want to be like, and attempt to imitate him or her. We even push our friends and relatives to be like this ideal and reach that other person's level. The efforts needed to achieve this goal often turn out to be unjustified and harmful for us and our friends and families.

So don't try to imitate anyone. You should find yourself and strive to develop yourself in accordance with your abilities. The desire to be better than others at any cost is stupid and destructive. It is like chasing the wind.

Example 2

Many have an excessive attachment to money, relationships with friends and family, things you own, your career or social status, etc. It is wrong to belittle the value of these things for human life, but it is also wrong to make the price we pay for achieving these goals or obtaining these things excessive. Nature teaches us that there is a balance in all things. These values must be of secondary importance.

If our relationships with friends and family deteriorate, if our material or social status drops, if our career is in danger, etc., and we are too attached to these things, the nervous stress can become severe enough to cause serious illness or even death.

When we cling to all these values, we do not account for the most important of our values, our life, given to us by God. Life itself is the greatest of all our treasures. Yet it is precisely this treasure that we are most willing to sacrifice in order to preserve the other treasures mentioned above.

Example 3

When insults, slander, humiliation, treachery, injustice, etc., are taken to heart—especially when they come from people we know well or care about (which is usually the case)—they are even more destructive for us.

94

Our usual reaction to such a situation is to decide that the person who insulted us is bad and insulted us unjustly. For a long time, we carry the offence in ourselves and imagine bad thoughts about them, including revenge. These emotions are destructive and can bring serious diseases.

Instead of automatically assuming that the other person is the problem, consider that the offence may have been because in our behavior there is something that needs to be corrected. Some people can not only see our problem in our words and actions, but can also read it at the subconscious level. Then they use one means or another to try to correct us, that is, teach us a lesson that would change us for the better, or make us review our opinion of someone or something, or save us from something worse.

If you recognize this, you will handle this "offence" as an opportunity to check yourself, and not necessarily as an assault on you personally. Once you realize this, you should not feel injured or imagine plans of revenge. Such plans are emotional violence which only you will feel. The other person will not feel this violence. You are hurting only yourself.

Think about it this way. If what he or she said is true, then you can turn it to your benefit through careful self-examination and fixing that problem. Even if a dyed-in-the-wool, genuine enemy criticizes you honestly and truthfully he or she has served you as a friend by pointing out a deficiency. Once you have repaired the problem, you are stronger.

If what he or she said is false, and you realize it after careful consideration, then you have benefitted by doing a healthy self-check on that topic. If one person thought it, perhaps some "fine-tunes" are in order even if you are not really guilty.

Even if he or she is wrong, protect yourself from the emotional violence hurled at you by forgiving. True forgiveness comes from the heart, and is 100%. Once you have truly forgiven, the violence vaporizes and can no longer harm you physically, emotionally, or spiritually. The Bible says, "Turn the other cheek."

How to Receive the Support of God

When faced with a serious problem, one that is more serious than a mere insult, many people turn to God for wisdom and help. Doing so is the First Wisdom.

However, do not ignore help from your friends, co-workers, professionals, or yourself. God gave you a brain. Use it. He also provided the many people who fill your life. This is a great resource. The Bible teaches, "There is wisdom in many counselors." The greatest treasures are sometimes hidden in plain view. Seek help from others. You will be surprised at how many people have been through the same thing or something similar, or they know others who have successfully dealt with your problem or issue.

Be grateful for the many resources you have at hand. Being grateful is as healing as true forgiveness.

Remember, if you are kind, considerate, and you know how to apply, God can help you with many complicated problems, but you need to understand, as stated by one famous Indian philosopher, "God has no other hands except your hands."

God's power resides inside of each individual, and if you apply rightly to God, praying, cleansing, correcting your diet, doing exercise and relaxation, living in kindness and forgiveness, this power will wake up and help you to solve many health and life problems.

96

Testimonials

How I Found My Perfect Diet

I love to read literature on health and do a lot of research on the subject. When I read about vegetarian diet, I liked the idea of not eating dead animals and eat live products instead. However, when I refused meet, I began craving sweets (for some balance and satisfaction), which I began eating for desert in each meal and even in between. Doing so, damaged my digestion, gave me yeast infections, frequent colds, sinus problems and allergies.

So I refused the vegetarian diet and learned about Atkins diet. In the beginning it felt fine and seemed to be working. However, after a few months I got sick of so much meet consumption. I also began feeling discomfort in my joints and kidneys. My flexibility got worse as well.

Then I heard wonders about all raw diet. I went through a course of how to "cook" raw food and was very enthusiastic about the idea. I didn't understand then that not everything raw is healthy, that not everything can be mixed together and especially did not realize the importance of hygiene for raw products. Nobody taught me this either. As a result, in a few months— bloated abdomen like a drum, indigestion and constant discomfort in my stomach.

Some luck brought me to Dr. Koyfman. In his center, I cleansed all my internal organs: colon, small intestine, stomach, liver, etc. Immediately I felt much better, my energy improved, my abdomen feels light and looks flat, my mood is much better. Dr. Koyfman helped me realize that we are all different and it is very important to find an individual diet that would work specifically for me. What I liked about Dr. Koyfman is that he helped me understand my body and its needs. He helped me balance my diet by eating variety of foods which agreed with my system and provided all the necessary nourishment. I've never felt better than now.

- Jordan. D , Tampa, FL

"My Diet Has Easily and Naturally Improved"

I had been trying to change my diet for many years without success—I was often tired, drank coffee daily, had severe PMS, and carried an extra 10-15 lbs. But somehow I just didn't have the willpower to make changes and take the time to prepare healthy foods.

Since starting Dr. Koyfman's "Eight Steps to Total Body Cleansing" my diet has easily and naturally improved . . . and the weight has fallen off! After just a few colonics, and feeling so much 'cleaner,' I automatically began to choose more raw, natural foods and even began juicing. I am now much more aware of when and how to eat (and drink!) And have no desire for many of the unhealthy foods I used to eat daily, especially sugar and animal protein.

With each cleansing procedure I go through at the Koyfman Center, I have more energy and am more aware of what different foods and diets can do to my body over time. I now eat less much more naturally and feel much better about eating generally. Dr. Koyfman's guidance overall and his nutrition information specifically I feel have definitely changed my life (and my family's eating habits) for the better forever! I am very grateful for his work and the efforts of his staff. Thank you!   —Linda Chmar,Atlanta, GA

"Making Sense of My Food Choices"

I distinctly remember my immense disappointment when, as a child, I first realized that a certain untasty, unwelcome dish of food was called plums. I had come to love plums during the previous summer, and I stood in astonishment that these could be the same thing. They were canned plums.

Further, I noticed that a fresh fruit that gave me energy and pleasure might, in a few months time, be very distasteful and upsetting to my system, so much so that I would stop buying that particular produce in the store.

You can tell I was pretty mixed up in my food choices. As a committed vegetarian, I sometimes despaired of eating well. I was also reaping physical consequences of these food choices in tensions, energy drain, and various pains.

Dr. Koyfman's reasoning has begun to make sense for me of the things I have felt and struggled with for a lifetime. The idea of eating in-season fruits and vegetables has taken the guessing out of what to buy at the store. The recognition that my body likes living food much better than dead food has helped me search for and discover things live and in season at most times of the year.

Dr. Koyfman's teaching does more than tell me what to do. It helps me learn to listen to my own body to know what is good or not good for me myself in each moment and place where I find myself. No one but I can make the choices for me, and I am grateful for all the wisdom I have learned at the Koyfman Center.

Now I choose food and eating habits that increase rather than steal my energy. I can tell when my body gains or loses by my choices. I can make informed decisions and live each day in vitality. Thank you, Dr. Koyfman.

—Wilma Zalabak, Atlanta, GA

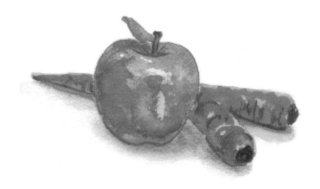

About our Cleansing Center

Philosophy and Services

The Immune System and Toxicity

Living today is hard on the body! Environmental poisons, food additives, stresses at home and at work, plus a wide diversity of other stresses come together to overload the body's resources. Resulting tensions, wastes, parasites, and many illnesses which thrive in such conditions produce poisons throughout the body. These are the poisons that weaken the body on its way to the grave.

God created within the body its own cleansing organs and systems (colon, kidneys, skin, lungs, lymph) which work to eradicate the incoming toxins. This system is both brilliant and powerful. To ignore it is to short circuit the wisest physician you can ever have working for you.

However, this system is not perfect. Bringing the power of the mind to work with this system can increase its effectiveness immensely. This is done when the mind realizes the wonderful array of cleansing techniques available to the body. It also happens when good nutritional practices are implemented.

There is another consideration. Each person's body has different strengths and weaknesses. For example, one person's liver is powerful while another's is not. Conversely, the person with a weaker liver has a stronger colon. The permutations on this are endless, and are due to genetic makeup, lifestyle and personal history. Because of this tremendous individuality in strengths and weaknesses, professionals trained in natural health care and cleansing are a powerful ally and weapon in the fight for optimal health.

Since the body gradually accumulates more and more stored toxins, which continue to poison their host, the immune system, driven to neutralize the effects of the stored poisons, becomes overworked and weakened.

As life goes on, the toxins accumulate to the extent that they create blockages in one or several vital channels such as arteries and other blood vessels, liver ducts, kidneys, breathing passages, or the digestive tract. These blockages have become the major causes of death in today's world.

Good diet, proper exercise, and healthy lifestyle can reduce incoming toxins and increase outgoing toxins, but they cannot stop the accumulation. Toxins do continue to enter and accumulate, coming as they do, not only from food, but also from environmental and other sources beyond our control and common to our daily lives.

One way to reduce the toxicity in the body to a level that is not dangerous, and then to maintain this level, is to use cleansing procedures.

What Are Cleansing Procedures?

Cleansing procedures are specifically designed to help the body eliminate accumulated waste and poison from internal organs, vital channels, and cells. Any treatment of illness will not yield long-term health improvement if these toxins are not eliminated from the body. Cleansing procedures do this work quickly and effectively.

Cleansing procedures in our Center use only natural means and methods. Clean water, herbs, fresh juices, massage of internal organs, heat, and special solutions help to dissolve the wastes and poisons stored in the various organs. Our Center's state-of-the-art cleansing and massage equipment serves to protect and enhance the natural processes of the body. This includes equipment to perform lymph drainage, lymph node cleansing, sinus cleansing, heavy metals elimination, and an infrared sauna.

How Soon Can a Person Feel Better with These Procedures?

Everything is individualized. One person may find some improvement after the first procedure. In other cases, it takes more time. One thing that anyone and everyone agrees on is that the removal of poisons, toxins, and wastes from the body will improve one's health.

What Procedures Does a Person Need?

The beginning of any cleansing program requires colon cleansing, as consideration of this picture will illustrate.

What's Wrong With This Picture?

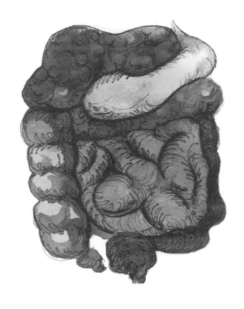

The colon depicted here is suffering from being stuffed with undigested food, toxic mucus, fermenting wastes, putrefied feces, and gas that has a similar toxic chemical composition.

A colon thus *expanded* with old fecal matter, gas, and new food puts pressure on neighboring organs. This pressure can hinder and sometimes seriously block the circulation of fluids in, to and around these organs. This interferes with the natural removal of wastes, and the delivery of oxygen and nutrients.

103

Chemically, such a wretched colon has the necessary environmental (anaerobic) conditions for starting and supporting all kinds of unwanted biological organisms, such as parasites, worms, viruses, and bacteria. Toxins stuck to the colon wall are absorbed through the colon walls, and spread to other organs and systems all over the body. Once in their new home or repository they form either toxic mucous or crystals the size of sand or small stones. These then become problems that poison and weaken the system further.

This same kind of process has been found operating in the arteries, veins, and other passages throughout the body. Plaque building up on the walls of blood vessels and arteries is one of the more famous examples of this basic process. This makes the heart's work more difficult and translates to feelings of tiredness and fatigue.

For prevention, our Center recommends cleansing of the large intestine or colon, followed by a systematic cleansing of the major organs. Parasite cleansing would complete the basic program. Once the vast majority of the body's organs are cleansed, a maintenance program would be part of the healthy lifestyle.

To solve a specific health problem, we can tailor an individualized program which will include cleansing procedures (such as Stomach Cleansing, Cleansing the Whole Digestive System, Small Intestine Cleansing, Liver Cleansing, etc.), diet, exercise, and other components necessary to creating a healthy lifestyle. The more serious the problem, the more time is required.

Proof of the benefit of the cleansing procedures may be seen after the first to fifth cleansing procedures. You will begin to feel better and have more energy. Your immune system will become stronger. Gradually the problem will become less, and for many people it will disappear.

In our Center the client also receives education in right eating, healthy recipes, cleansing exercises, and the healthy lifestyle.

Dr. Yakov Koyfman, Naturopathic Doctor

As early as 1976, Dr. Koyfman was interested in alternative medicine in Ukraine, Russia. His first experiments were on himself, as he helped his own sinus and digestive problems, back pain, and colds. Then he did extensive study and self-research under famous doctors from India, Russia, and Japan. He studied nutrition, dietology, and fasting therapy in Russia. He is certified by the American (and Georgia State) Naturopathic Medical Association. He is certified also by the International Association for Colon HydroTherapy (I.-A.C.T.). He holds a diploma as a European and Oriental Massage Therapist (First Degree), and a diploma from the National Board of Naturopathic Examiners. His system combines experience, knowledge, and techniques from the East and from the West.

In 1994, Dr. Koyfman founded his Center in America, and has helped thousands of people since then. People come for help from not only Atlanta, but also from other states and countries including Florida, Washington, and New York, Canada, Germany, Israel, and Russia.

Dr. Koyfman has authored many articles and books where he describes his health philosophy. You can order these books from the Center, or buy them in some health food stores. Note: The following article was published in *Natural Awakenings, Atlanta Edition,* October, 2002, pages 26-27. The interviewer, Wilma Zalabak, M.Div., is consultant for the

Koyfman Center and president of The Atlanta Listenary at www.listenary.com.

Health & Cleansing: An Interview with Dr. Yakov Koyfman, N.D.

WZ: Dr. Koyfman, you have a wide base of training and experience in helping people to fight disease and gain health. What would you say is the basic cause which destroys our health and leads to disease?

Dr. K: I am practically sure that the first cause of all disease is toxicity.

Toxicity is the result of a poor diet and an unhealthy lifestyle. In a polluted body, the immune system constantly fights with toxins. As a result of this fight the body's defense becomes weaker. Bacteria, viruses, and parasites start growing in toxicity without resistance from a weakened immune system. These scavengers steal the best nutrients from the system. They consume nutrients from food, blood, cells, and organs. Besides stealing nutrients, they excrete additional toxins into the system.

WZ: So, you claim that toxicity alone is the single cause of all health problems? Or have we another situation which may destroy our health?

Dr. K: We have other powerful reasons for illnesses in negative emotions, stresses, and depressions. When we get nervous or stressed, we automatically close down and tighten muscles, nerves, and vital organs. As a result, these strong emotions record themselves as cell memories and remain as constant tensions in the muscles and internal organs. In tight areas of organs, there is destruction of blood and lymph circulation, digestion, nervous system, etc., and these conditions create blockages in these areas. All this leads to new toxicity in the system. Even the best food eaten during stress changes to toxins. In reacting to a stress situation, an unclean system is much more sensitive than a clean body. Let me point to four basic reasons which lead to various diseases: **pollution in the body, parasites, nutrient deficiency, and stress.** In natural medicine we look for cure, not to the doctor, but to nature. Our main goal is prevention and improving the immune system.

WZ: What is the link between the immune system and toxicity?

Dr. K: A clean body has a strong immune system, able to fight well with different health disorders. The greater the power of the immune system the greater the level of the person's health. To improve the immune system one must eliminate toxins, bacteria, and parasites from the system which disturb the body's own self-healing efforts.

Alternative medicine always tries to eliminate the root of illness and not just the symptoms. It fights, not against nature, but together with nature. It heals the system and helps to restore health by eliminating toxic substances and changing the lifestyle.

WZ: Dr. Koyfman, Some people are afraid to do colon cleansing, thinking that this procedure may flush friendly bacteria from their colon. What is your opinion?

Dr. K: Many people don't seem afraid to put into their systems dangerous and even poisonous beverages and food, but they are afraid to cleanse this junk from their systems. When we do cleansing, we eliminate toxins and dangerous bacteria from the system but not friendly flora. In a polluted system there are practically no friendly flora. After cleansing, if you eat right and take acidophilus, you will begin growing friendly bacteria in your system.

Here is one example: A world famous American doctor, Norman Walker, when he got sick at age 50, had no fear of flushing friendly bacteria from his system. He did colon cleansing every week for the rest of his life. He lived a long and healthy life to 119 years. When he was 102 years old, he fathered a daughter.

WZ: What makes your Center different from others?

Dr K: In our Center we do, not just colon cleansing, which is a very important procedure (I call it the first step to health), but also other cleansings which I have named **total body cleansing.** Total body cleansing includes cleansing the colon, stomach, small intestines, gall bladder, pancreas, lungs, kidneys, liver, blood vessels, sinuses, and more. We also educate people in how to rid themselves of negative emotions. We teach them exercises which can help them improve the cleansing process and gain more energy. We pay lots of attention to healthy diet.

This brings to our Center we clients, not only from Atlanta, Georgia, but also from other cities and states like Boston, Virginia, Florida, California, and sometimes even from other countries.

WZ: I think the readers will be interested to know what health problems people bring to your Center and how your cleansing procedures may help them.

Dr. K: I will give a few **more** examples without names, for confidentiality reasons.

A woman, 43 years old, suffered for two years from constant cough, allergies, and asthma. She was treated by many doctors with tons of medicine without favorable results. After a month of our cleansing program, the cough had completely stopped, and her medicine was discarded in the trash. After two months, she was free from asthma and allergy.

A man, around 40 years old, had prostate tumors, intense pain, and difficulty in urination, with an abnormal blood test. Doctors urged him to have an operation. After a month of cleansing procedures, the pain was completely gone. After four months, the tumor had disappeared and the blood test was normal. He looked 10-15 years younger than his age.

A woman, 48 years old, had high blood pressure, frequent depression, and complaints of constant fatigue. She carried 40 pounds of excess weight. After a month of cleansing, her blood pressure became normal. After three months, she was full of energy and depression was gone. After six months, she looked like a model.

Such examples come by the hundreds. The youngest of our clients is a little more than five years old, and the oldest is almost 100 years old.

WZ: Dr. Koyfman, do you know a universal method for being healthy and living a long life?

Dr. K: The universal method for being healthy is a healthy lifestyle.

Every day we take a shower to cleanse our body and get rid of its smell. Several times each day we wash our hands and face, brush our teeth, moisturize our lips, and comb our hair, but we do nothing at all to take care of our internal organs, glands, vessels, etc. Many of us don't even know where they are located even though, in many ways, our health depends on the health of our internal organs, glands, and nervous system.

In addition to not paying attention to our organs and glands, we have such a lifestyle that destroys them and leads to disease. When our organs get ill and feel pain, the pain we feel is because these sick organs are our organs. We run to the doctor to get drugs, to shut down their voice so as not to hear their cries for help.

If we want to be healthy, we have to lead a healthy lifestyle and take care of our internal organs, cleansing them and improving their strength the same as we take care of our hands, skin, hair, etc.

A healthy lifestyle means regularly cleansing the body on a deep level as we do in our Center. A healthy lifestyle also means every day helping your organs to cleanse themselves through things you can do by yourself: choosing a healthy diet, exercising to improve the strength of your internal organs, cleansing your body from negative emotions, and other self-cleansing procedures. Usually people overlook what is in their lifestyle about diet, thoughts, emotions. These things play a vital role in either destroying or improving health.

At the same time, in order to be healthy, your internal organs need constant daily support. Every day you need to help your body to cleanse the large intestine, the kidneys, the lungs, the skin, the liver, etc.

Every day you need to help your body to cleanse the blood vessels, the blood, the lymph, and the thyroid gland.

The thyroid gland plays and important role in the defense of your body. It is the main fortress in your system. Every day you need to maintain good blood circulation in the brain to restore a right connection between the brain and other internal organs. This connection is constantly being broken by negative thoughts and emotions. The lack of a proper connection between the brain and the internal organs leads to health disorders.

Every day you need to help your sex organs to restore proper circulation and to cleanse themselves from toxicity. Sex organ disease has become an epidemic which threatens the health- and even lives of women and men.

Every day, you need to feed your body vital food and also help your digestive organs convert this food into nutrients, not poisons. When you ignore the principles of healthy eating, even the best foods and supplements will create toxicity.

All these secrets, which I have gained in 25 years of practice, and many other useful devices, I describe in my books, *Deep Internal Body Cleansing, Eight Steps to Perfect Health, Unique Method of Colon Rejuvenation,* and *Healing through Cleansing, Books 1-4.*

When I wrote these books, I tried to follow two main tasks: (1) I tried to give simple, practical, and effective methods which really work to improve and maintain health. (2) I tried to describe things clearly and persuasively so everybody who reads them can understand and be inspired with the desire to do what is described.

Everybody can find in these books the answer to that question that is most important and what he or she needs to learn to help the body restore and maintain health through simple and natural methods. If somebody needs further consultation or help, in our Center we are always happy to help. We also work in cooperation with medical doctors who

111

have opened their mind and understand that health depends, not on medicine, but on the individual's own efforts coupled with professional guidance.

Our Center can recommend the following books to help guide you down the path of optimum health.

1. How to help clean your organs with professional help is described in my books: *Deep Internal Body Cleansing,* and *Eight Steps to Perfect Health.*

2. How to help your own system through self-help methods is described in my books, *Healing through Cleansing, Books 1-4,* and *Unique Method of Colon Rejuvenation.*

To learn more about unique cleansing procedures done in our center, please visit our website at

w w w . k o y f m a n c e n t e r . c o m

Unique Method of Colon Rejuvenation, 95 pages; $12.

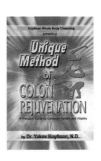

Our bodies need constant help eliminating toxic substances which enter the system every day. Daily practice of the rising and restroom exercises described in this book strengthens colon muscles so that, with time, elimination will accompany each meal and eject more toxins than are retained. Also included are principles and recipes for healthy eating, raw meals, and safe cooking technology.

Eight Steps to Total Body Cleansing and Perfect Health, 214 pages; $20.

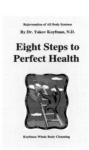

You will find here how to prepare for cleansing and what to expect during Deep Internal Body Cleansing. You will want to know what to do if you feel any discomfort during the cleansing. This book explains how we perform Deep Internal Body Cleansing at the Center. Also, you will discover here what to eat after the cleansing in order to maintain your success and your new lifestyle.

Deep Internal Body Cleansing, 172 pages. $15

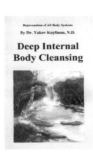

If you search for healing and real health, then here you will find answers to your questions Here is information about toxicity and the immune system, healthy eating and eliminating parasites. Here are answers to help you resist hurtful cravings and negative emotions. You really can get health and gain energy through cleansing your body.

Healing Through Cleansing - Book 1, 114 pages; $12.

Every day, toxic substances enter our bodies from the various chemical and biological contaminants in our environment. Additionally, toxins form within us due to poor dietary habits, stress, aging, and harmful bacteria that populate our bodies. Our excretory organs can't cope with such a large amount of work and need constant, conscious support. How can you help your main excretory organs become free of toxins, bacteria, and 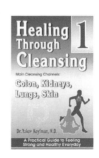 infections? You will find the answers in the pages of this and subsequent books in this Koyfman Series.

Healing Through Cleansing - Book 2, 101 pages; $12.

In many ways our health depends on the health of organs located in the head and neck regions: the brain, thyroid gland, eyes, salivary glands, ears, nose and sinuses, throat, tongue, teeth and gums. The contemporary American diet usually includes a large number of mucus-forming foods that result in the generation of mucus throughout the body. Excess mucus settles throughout the body, especially in the head and neck organs, giving rise to a number of ailments in these organs.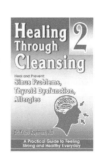

Healing Through Cleansing - Book 3, 120 pages; $12.

The abdominal area is the kitchen of our bodies. How well or poorly this kitchen functions depends on whether we feed our system with nutrients or poison our system with toxicity. If your abdominal kitchen produces nutrients, you are getting health; if your kitchen produces poison, you are getting disease.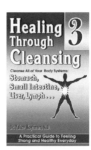